CAREGIVING TIPS
A-Z

by Starr Calo-oy
with Bob Calo-oy

Alzheimer's & Other Dementias

D1120926

★ *Starr Calo-oy* ★

CAREGIVING TIPS A-Z
Alzheimer's & Other Dementias
by Starr & Bob Calo-oy

Meet Cappy & Daisy!

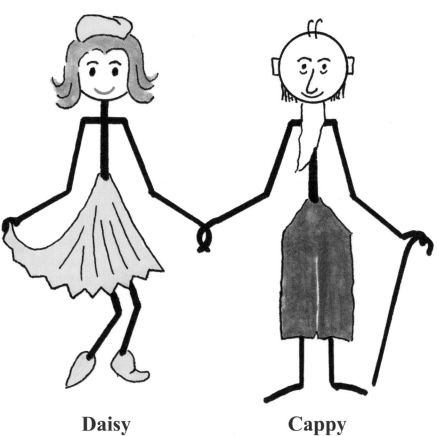

Daisy
(caregiver/daughter)

Cappy
(Dad)

Caregiving Tips A-Z
Alzheimer's & Other Dementias
by Starr & Bob Calo-oy

Published by Orchard Publications
P.O. Box 680815
San Antonio, Texas 78268
www.caregiversadvice.net

Copyright 2008 by Starr Calo-oy
First Edition 2008
ISBN # 978-0-9753195-3-6
Printed in the United States of America

(1) Caregiving (2) Caregivers (3) Sandwich generation (4) Behavioral problems (5) Aging Parents (6) Elderly (7) Elder health (8) Alzheimer's Disease (9) Baby boomers (10) Care Tips (11) Seniors

This publication is sold with the understanding that the publisher and authors are not engaged in rendering professional advice. A physician should be consulted before adopting any of the suggestions in this book. The authors and publisher disclaim any liability arising directly or indirectly from the use of this book.

All Illustrations in this book are by Dr. Charles A. Belfi.

CONTENTS

THANK YOU, THANK YOU, THANK YOU!!!!

We are a product of our experiences and those people who have crossed our paths. I am blessed to have met some of the finest people in the world.

Unless you have gone through the process of writing a book, you can't imagine how much support is required from those in your life in order to complete it. This is the reason you will see a page or two like this one at the beginning of most books. I am so thankful, as an author, to many people, and certainly, the following.

I acknowledge, appreciate and deeply care about the people who have stood by me to complete not only this book, but also its companion, *"Caregiving Tips A-Z, Alzheimer's & Other Dementias."*

Thank you, my precious Bob, for protecting my strict writing schedule, making sure all my needs were met, having undying and unselfish patience with all of my moods, helping me unlock the words in my mind that were struggling to get out and above all, for loving me unconditionally. I love you.

Thank you, Charles, for always being there for me, putting yourself last to help me meet my unending goals, stretching your artistic borders to illustrate our books, sacrificing your goals, time and sleep to get the job done and constantly showing your love in a million ways on a daily basis.

Thank you, Daddy (Bob Turner), for always believing in me, encouraging me, being such an amazing man and father and being so strong in every way and for taking such good care of our mother.

Thank you to Khaiyan & Khalea (our smallest children), for giving me the time I needed to write. I know you missed being with me. I love you so much. If it weren't for your patience, I never could have finished these two books or any of the others.

Thank you, my sisters, Debi Ursell and Janiece Hartman and our brother, Bob Turner Jr. for walking with me through and helping me with our mothers' graduation to heaven. Your love sustained me.

Thank you, Jacqueline Marcell, for writing such a well-written and heartfelt foreword to both of my latest books. I am humbled by your writing (*Elder Rage*) and consider it a great honor to have your stamp of approval on mine.

Thank you, Elva Garza, for sharing your most intimate triumph as a real life hero in the life of your mother, Lucia. You are a wonderful Christian woman.

Thank you our dear Friend, Albert Garza, for helping Bob and filling in the gap as our administrator. You are a Godsend and a brilliant businessman.

Thank you Hugo (Juice) Hinojosa, our personal assistant, for the long, late hours you work without ever complaining. You end the day with the same speed, strength and efficiency as you begin with and continually with a smile! We can always depend on you.

Thank you, once again, Mark Mayfield (Litho Press). You always save the day with your expertise, compassion, patience and artistic input. You are much more to us than our printer; you are our forever Friend.

Foreword

As our elderly population multiplies along with the escalating high cost of care, the thirst for more eldercare knowledge rises too. I believe the best source for teaching this hands-on information comes from devoted caregivers who have already "been there--done that". And yes, it is often helpful to hear healthcare professionals talk about how to be an effective caregiver, but it is quite another thing to actually *be* a caregiver.

Starr has truly earned her caregiving credibility by caring for the terminally ill (well-minded and those with Alzheimer's), as well as her own family members, in her own home for *eighteen* years! I have a special place in my heart for caregivers like Starr, who become so compelled by their experience they just have to share what they have struggled so hard to figure out-- and often learned "the hard way."

Instead of continuing to counsel families in person, Starr decided to start writing to bring the plight of caregivers to the world's consciousness. Her goal has been realized again here in her marvelous third book, "Caregiving Tips A-Z, Alzheimer's & Other Dementias". It's well researched and down-to-earth, with a gambit of valuable and practical advice on medical, physical, financial and emotional issues—all shared with heartfelt empathy assuring us we are not alone.

I fully understand Starr's need to share her hard-won

knowledge, because after the heart-wrenching experience of caring for my elderly parents (both with early Alzheimer's not properly diagnosed for over a year), I gave up my stalled career as a television executive to become an advocate for eldercare awareness and reform.

I too felt compelled to write a book, "Elder Rage", about my once-adoring father who turned abusive toward me, yet could act completely normal in front of the doctors when he needed to. It was an unbelievable nightmare, as I also fought through an unsympathetic medical system, but with sheer determination I solved the endless crisis medically and behaviorally. Ohhh, if I'd only had Starr's books to guide me then!

We need to realize that soon there will be more seniors alive than any other age group--and at any other time in history. The first wave of 76 million Baby Boomers (those born between 1946 and 1964) will begin turning sixty-five in 2011, but one in eight will be afflicted with dementia. And nearly half will be afflicted by age 85, the fastest growing age group because of medical technology.

How on earth will they all be taken care of when there is such a shortage of geriatric professionals, nurses and caregivers now? And where will the funds come from as Medicare and Medicaid get depleted? Part of the solution is knowledge and education for *everyone*—and Starr has provided our textbooks.

Starr, I want to congratulate you on this book and your many outstanding achievements! I am delighted we are comrades in the crusade to educate caregivers, especially those struggling to care for and keep at home--those suffering from dementia.

--Jacqueline Marcell
Best-selling author of "*Elder Rage*" and
host of the "Coping with Caregiving" radio program

PLEASE NOTE

1. FOR THE SAKE OF SIMPLICITY, WE HAVE CHOSEN TO REFER TO YOUR ELDERLY LOVED ONE IN THIS BOOK AS "LO."

2. FOR THE SAKE OF SPACE AND REDUNDANCY, WE HAVE CHOSEN TO USE THE WORDS:

   - "HE, HIM AND HIS" RATHER THAN "HE/HER" ETC. IF YOUR LO IS A FEMALE, ALL TIPS APPLY EQUALLY

   - "AD" FOR ALZHEIMER'S DISEASE

Introduction
"The Unsung Hero"

Beyond a doubt, the most noble endeavor, is one in which a person lays down his life, and everything that goes with it, to provide complete care for another human being. If you are a caregiver, you are to be praised.

Unless someone has been responsible for the very life of someone else; their sustenance, hygiene and health, they cannot imagine the weight of accountability to God that rests on their shoulders. If you are a caregiver, you are to be admired.

No one will ever see all the diapers you change, the showers you give, the mountains of laundry you wash or the never-ending messes you clean up daily. No one will ever know the full extent of the great sacrifices you have made; your privacy, time, energy, social life and career that you have surrendered for your LO. Even if you care for others outside your family as a career, most of the time, it's a thankless job and you will never get paid enough for it.

You should take holy pride in the fact that it was you who stepped up to the plate to care for your LO above all others who could have. God has called you to this great work and as someone once said "God doesn't call the qualified; He qualifies the called."

With the proper caregiving tools, knowledge to apply them and an open mind, this great calling can be made much easier. We hope to give you these tools in this book.

When an elderly LO has deteriorated in his health to the point that he must move in with one of his adult children, many

1

lives are changed forever.

Marriages become tested. Relationships with your children still living with you will go through the fire. Your sleep cycle will change. You will discover a new side of your relatives. You will get to know the real you better than you ever have before. But, when you finally get to bed at night, you will experience the greatest satisfaction in knowing that you have provided hands-on care with a loving touch that only you could provide.

One day, when the young seed of your youth has grown into a mature oak tree in the autumn of your life, you will reap the care you have sown into your LO.

During the course of our 18 years of professional caregiving in our own home, Bob and I were privileged to take care of my Branny and my mother until they passed away. I can't tell you how satisfying it was for me to provide relief to their pain and put their fears to rest. I loved serving them and my entire family. Helping my siblings and my dad through the journey of their passing was indescribably fulfilling.

While mother was in the hospital, each evening Bob and I would spend several hours there. With the curtain pulled and Bob reading on one side of it, I spent priceless time with her. I bathed her gently and then gave her a full-body massage with scented oils and lotions. She looked so forward to our arrival each day.

Words cannot express the fulfillment I experienced as I rubbed the oil into her skin, knowing how much it meant to her. I now rejoice because although I knew she was dying and I could not do anything to prevent it, I made her last two months on Earth very comfortable. I made her feel pampered and loved. We all did. She was surrounded by those she loved most and who adored her.

Before we'd leave, I would change her bedding and gown, prop her up with four pillows, pray with her and kiss her good night. I slept so well at night because of this and so did she.

When she came to our home for care after the hospitalization, we continued our nightly ritual. It was "our time." Touch took on a whole new meaning.

We provided loving care for our elderly for 18 years, but this was my own mother now and she made it clear that she wanted to be with me. She trusted my care. This was a great honor. Mother went on to live with Jesus in August of 2006.

I share this with you because as you read our books, keep in mind that I don't write from a clinical or head-knowledge point of view. I write from my heart, in addition to a wealth of experience, because I've been there too.

I understand the emotional minefields in watching a LO struggle to hold on to life. I understand the weight of caregiving. I understand how you feel and want you to know that you are not alone. I may not know you but I am very, very proud of you for undertaking the unselfish care of your LO, even if no one else tells you this.

Your LO may not be able to express how much he appreciates you, but be assured of this: God sees everything you are doing, every sacrifice you make and He smiles at the mention of your name. He is proud of you.

You are an unsung hero among those who walk the Earth. You are my hero and I dedicate this book to you.

Starr Calo-oy

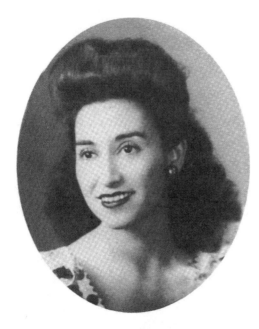

Young Lucia Anguiano

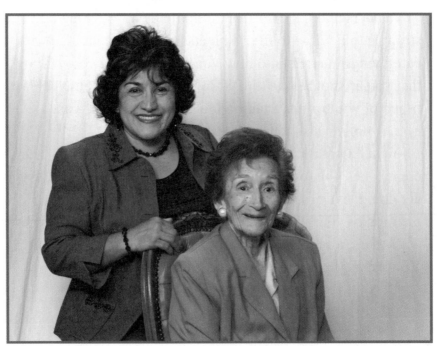

Elva and Lucia

Portrait of a Hero
Daughter, Elva Garza
(Of thee I sing)

Who would imagine, while driving down Callaghan Road in San Antonio, Texas, a modern day hero was quietly working in her home, doing what heroes do?

State Farm agent by day and super hero by (day and) night, meet Elva Garza; an amazing woman, wife, mother and daughter.

Many of you will be able to easily identify with the elements of her personal story. Much of this story has to do with Elva's upbringing. I am compelled to share it with you.

Elva's mother, Lucia Anguiano, was born April 27, 1917 in Poteet, Texas to migrant workers. Every summer, her parents would travel to Michigan in the big trucks with her four sisters and three brothers, to pick cherries and beans in the fields.

Elva was born in San Antonio, Texas to Ismael (Smiley) & Lucia Aguilar on November 24, 1950.

Although Lucia only had a third grade education, she held the highest standards, teaching her children about Jesus all their lives. Her parents and grandparents were very active in the Baptist church, so it followed that Elva and her sister, Lucy, were also.

When Elva was one and a half years old, Lucia divorced and raised her children in the deep west side as a single parent. She never remarried.

Lucia, her two daughters and Camilla and her five children

all lived together in a very modest home that had been in the family for many years. Lucia's brother and sister-in-law (Abel & Lola) and their nine children lived next door to them in another small home which also belonged to the family.

While Lucia worked to support the family, Abel & Lola raised their own children and took care of Elva and Lucy, her sister.

Elva recalls that even though she thought they were poor, her aunt and her children had it much worse. Lucia always taught the children "If we only have one tortilla left in the house, we will share it with your aunt and the other kids."

Lucia taught her family the meaning of sacrificial love and they learned well. The Lord always made ends meet somehow. Her sowing kindness and generosity into others less fortunate was also apparent in the way she handled her vacations.

While other employees went off to vacation somewhere else, Lucia would be found using hers to serve at vacation bible school. Later, she would work in the nursery at church and watch her grandchildren so that Elva could serve in numerous church duties as she once did.

Elva left home in 1973 to get married but divorced after 6 years.

Lucia worked at Esskay Manufacturing Company, to provide for her family, as a trimmer, hemming men's pants. On the weekends, she'd do laundry, cook for the week and clean. She was Elva's babysitter, helping her to realize her dream as a successful businesswoman.

Elva reciprocated by not attending Baylor University because her mother didn't want her to leave San Antonio.

Instead, she attended St. Mary's University and graduated in 1973.

In 1979, the adult children in the family decided to sell Lucia's house because it was literally falling apart. By that time, all of the children were adults and had moved on. The same year, after Elva's divorce, Lucia moved back in to care for the children after school and on weekends while still holding down a full time job.

Elva became a State Farm agent in April of 1981. She fondly remembers the aroma of fresh menudo, caldo and calabasita as her mother cooked in the back part of her office.

Lucia was still working at that time but retired in 1983. Elva remarried in 1987. This man, Albert Garza, was (and is) her knight in shining armor. He not only married Elva; he married her mother too! He has always been there for all of Elva's family and extremely patient and understanding about the special relationship between her and her mother. Lucia was always a little jealous of Albert. She was worried that he would whisk Elva away from her and she'd be left alone, but that would never happen.

Up until May of 2001, Lucia had been completely independent; dressing up, driving her own car and shopping by herself. But that month, everything changed.

Lucia was never one to take a daytime nap but Elva found her asleep at 1:30 p.m. when she had returned home to check in. She knew instantly that something was wrong with her mother. She shook her frantically.

The doctor said Lucia had suffered a TIA (small brain stroke) and that if Elva had not roused her, she would probably been paralyzed. You really couldn't tell she had a stroke except that her face on one side was sagging a bit.

Lucia drove only six more months and that was against her doctor's wishes. There were great disagreements between them during that time about her driving. The doctor warned her that she could end up killing herself and others if she had another stroke while driving. He said she should never drive again.

Finally, Elva hid her mother's keys to keep her from driving but that still didn't stop her.

It was a Sunday afternoon in the latter part of 2002 and Lucia stayed home from church that day while Albert and Elva attended. The plan was that Lucia was to be ready for them to pick her up and take her out for lunch when church dismissed.

Elva called her mother saying "We should be home to get you in about ten minutes. What are you doing?"

Lucia said defiantly, "There is no reason for you to come get me. Go ahead and go to lunch without me. I'm eating my tamales."

Elva's heart sank as she said, "Did someone bring them to you?" Her mother said, "No! I took my car and went and got my own tamales! I can drive better than the two of you!" Elva lost her appetite and went home. There was her mother- sitting at the table with a cup of coffee and a dozen tamales!

It was that day when Elva and Albert decided to sell her car which made her mother extremely upset with them and later on, become depressed. Elva suffered tremendous mixed emotions. She wanted mother to maintain her independence while at the same time, was trying to protect her from hurting herself.

From 2002-2005, her mother was still able to dress and

groom herself with no assistance. Elva had to take her mother to run her errands, go to doctor visits and all the places Lucia was used to going by herself.

In 2005, Elva had to take over bathing her mother and helping to toilet her. Lucia was very upset that her privacy was intruded upon, but Elva knew she could easily slip, fall and break a bone if left to herself. Lucia fought her the first few times but finally conceded.

In 2006, the family began noticing drastic changes. Lucia, then 89 years old, no longer cared about her appearance or matching her clothes. She began shadowing Elva like a little, lost puppy, following her around everywhere.

Lucia continually paces around saying it's time to go, regardless of where she is or how long she has been there. She cannot do anything for herself anymore.

Elva has grief, loss, pain, exhaustion, mixed emotions and a lot of love. As I said, you will probably identify with her.

Elva misses her mother dressing up each day and being on the go all the time. She misses seeing her drive off in her car. She misses the mommy in Lucia. The reversal of roles is very painful to live through, but Elva says that she is grateful to God that her mother is still alive.

Elva is a hero because she has made the decision to care for her mother regardless of inconvenience, personal sacrifice and has been with her mother for the past twenty-eight years showing her loving patience and loving-kindness. They have lived together for all but six years of Elva's entire life.

With all the tumultuous, mixed emotions, she remembers the mommy who taught her how to appreciate what she had, even though it was not much, and to share what she did have. She now gives back to her mother and to many others.

She doesn't wear a cape or disguise but if Lucia still had the presence of mind to articulate, she would tell you Elva is her superhero. The Lord sees her the same way.

Special Note:

While interviewing Elva for her story, she related to me that she wanted to share the names of her family who contributed to helping her over the years with Lucia. They are listed below.

Elva's children & grandchildren:

- Fernando (son) & wife, Rosemary Garza and their sons, Adriane & Andrew Garza
- Felina Hanlon (daughter), and her two daughters, Deanna & Melanie Hanlon
- Steven Joshua Morfin (son)

Lucy (Elva's sister) & Ernest Fernandez have one son; Ernest (Netito) Fernandez and his son, Javi Fernandez.

"Aging"
by Ray Cevallos

it is amazing how the years
go by so fast
why, there are less in my future
than there are in my past

but looking back at
all those years
i see a lot more laughter
than i see tears

oh, i feel sad for my brother and others
whose lives were short and never knew
the joy of hearing a grandchild whisper
momo , popo , i love you

and i learned that true happiness
comes from within
i can't tell you exactly where i'm going
but i can tell you where i've been

years ago my heart was broken
how can your heart not break when a child dies, it seems so wrong
yet that same broken heart would not quit
while battling a horrific cancer
it gave me compassion and made me strong

there is an aging man that lives in my mirror
who looks so much like my father
and i recall so vividly with reverence
the teachings and love of my mother

there are aches and pains and illnesses that come with aging
aging is a gift, so i am happy for me
because everyday i inch ever closer to being
the man that God, intended me to be

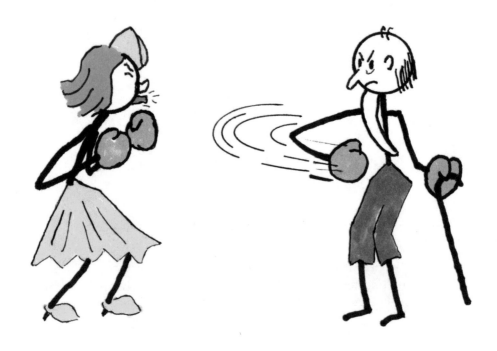

The Boxer

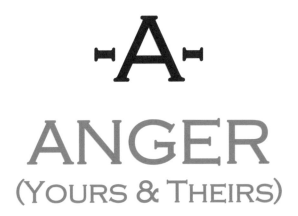

ANGER
(YOURS & THEIRS)

THIS CHAPTER:

- **Your Anger**
- **Your LO's Anger**

ANGER

(YOURS & HIS)

The most important truth you will need to accept when caring for a LO with dementia who leans toward exhibiting an angry behavior pattern, is that they truly have *no control* over their actions or the way they express their feelings. It may be very difficult for you to accept this, but you must if you eventually want peace.

If they were usually angry when their

mind was well, you may feel they are just being extra mean and stubborn now. You may only detect a small change at first and believe they are acting this way on purpose and could control their temper if given the proper incentive. You may try to lay a guilt trip on them, to no avail.

When dementia first begins to become apparent, the well-minded family member, not being able to see anything wrong physically, automatically believes their LO is faking it; that they are just trying to get attention. One of the reasons for this mistaken belief is that there are no physical manifestations of what is going on in their mind.

This is very unfortunate for both parties, as this misconception escalates into feelings of great anger in the family caregiver and confusion and fear for the person suffering with dementia.

If he was normally pleasant before, but now it seems as if his personality has changed, you may experience mixed emotions in your new perception of him. If a doctor informed you that he does indeed have dementia, then you must accept that you are dealing with an entirely different person who desperately needs your patience and kindness.

As we grow older, our patience diminishes and we tend to become more verbal about things that displease us or make us uncomfortable.

Almost everyone goes through this so it is important to keep in mind that one day; we will need the same grace and mercy from those younger than we are.

Whatever you do, do not react in anger or you will compound the problem and then feel guilty when all is said and done.

Before your own health starts to suffer,

please get in a support group and get some help, fast. You should also make an appointment to see your doctor for his advice and perhaps medication for you, as well as your pastor for prayerful support.

Do not make the mistake of thinking you are being brave and noble to carry all this on your shoulders; it could take your very life and then you will be of no help to your helpless LO at all.

Your Anger

You may have been together for 50, 60 or more years; you may be a spouse or an adult child. Do not be hard on yourself thinking, "I should be able to do this! I know my LO better than anyone does. Something must be wrong with me- I have to try harder."

Listed on the following pages are some ideas that have worked for us in the past. Do not give up. Keep trying different methods until you have successfully tasted sweet victory and then you will be proud of yourself.

PLAN OF ACTION
FOR YOUR ANGER!

TIP #1:

Call the Department of Human Services in your area and ask them where to get *"A Guide for Human Services"* for your state and send off for it.

When you get your guide, look up the word "abuse" and it will have a long list of sources for help along with their phone numbers. Do yourself and your LO a favor and make the calls.

So many people out there need help to control themselves when dealing with their LO as you do.

Do not be embarrassed. You should be proud of yourself for taking the first step. Please, get help before it is too late, you really hurt your LO, and you regret it for the rest of your life.

TIP #2:

If you are shoving and pushing out of anger, pinching, biting, scraping him with your fingernails, hitting or choking him or anything else you know in your heart qualifies as abuse, get someone to take care of your LO immediately and get away from him for the weekend. (See the chapter on "O" for Outside Help for suggestions)

When you get to the point that you are physically hurting the one you love, there is no other option other than seeking help for yourself and for him.

You may say to yourself, "This will be the last time I do this." These words are common with abuse so listen to yourself and recognize them.

TIP #3:

Make an appointment with your pastor. Be frank with him and ask for help in the way of a church support group and prayer. He can help you find your way.

If there is not a support group in your church, why not start one? There are many family caregivers secretly going through the same thing you are. As you move toward helping others, you automatically move toward healing yourself.

Only through forgiving yourself can you expect to start on the road to emotional recovery.

TIP #4:

It can be extremely frustrating to witness your LO grow old and become dependent on you.

There is a feeling of great loss and grief that occurs when the elder you have depended on all of your life for advice and help moves into a needy season. It can make you feel alone.

This may be where some of the anger you are feeling is coming from. Sharing these emotions with your siblings, who are probably struggling with the same sentiments, can help you to see things realistically. Share, grieve and laugh together and go on.

Instead of getting angry as you notice these changes, try a little mercy.

Remember, you will be old someday too and will

need your children to reach out to you instead of recoiling with disgust, anger and disappointment. You will reap what you sow. Sow well!

TIP #5:

Yelling, threatening, withholding things, cursing and throwing things are abuse too. You may be deceiving yourself that because you are not actually touching your LO when you get angry with him, that you are not abusing him. Do you think that a small, helpless child would agree with that?

TIP #6:

Call your local Alzheimer's Association, permanent placement facilities, such as personal care homes and nursing homes, for a list of

sitter's. They are a great resource whether your LO has Alzheimer's or not.

TIP #7:

The way we view our elderly, in today's day and age, has completely flip-flopped in comparison to biblical days when they were highly respected and revered.

In order to initiate a paradigm shift regarding your LO, ask him about his past experiences and really listen this time. You can learn so much about the world through his life and he will enjoy having someone to tell his story to.

If he has dementia and cannot relate the facts about his life, go through his photo albums with him and tell his story to him. Ask some other relatives to participate if they are willing.

The reasoning behind this exercise is that as you learn more about his life through other's eyes and their view of his opinions, thoughts and desires, you will not be so apt to lash out at him in anger.

You can more easily develop compassion and respect for one who has lived so much longer than you have and respect what he has been through. This will provide the paradigm shift you need to start responding instead of reacting.

TIP #8:

When you get to the point that you do not trust yourself to be alone with your LO, ask a friend or relative to temporarily move in with you. Even if they do not help with the day-to-day care, it is important for them to be with you to help keep you in check.

Accountability can help to change old life patterns. It takes a minimum of 30 days to establish a new life pattern to replace an old one. Consistency is key.

If you are too ashamed to disclose the reason why you need the company, do not feel you have to explain. The main issue is the safety of your LO.

Also, use caution with whom you share the intimate details of your actions. You do not need the ill judgment of others upon you right now. You need compassion and their help. If you feel you need to talk to someone, choose a person who is bound by confidentiality in their profession, such as a member of the clergy.

Tip #9:

Maybe you need reminding about "the good old days." Sometimes we get so caught up in the hands-on care and the daily routine that we lose sight of the wonderful memories we made together.

Get out the old, lose photos of your LO and put together a photo album chronicling his life; tell his story. This can help you get back in touch with the person he was the majority of his life and revive the respect you had for him before the dementia or difficult behavior became apparent.

It can also help you to gain some self-respect and help you to feel good about yourself again. Have your LO help you if they are able. If not, at least let them sit with you as you do it.

After you finish the album, you will have so much to talk about and the reminiscing will be very therapeutic for both of you.

Tip #10:

When **you** get "cabin fever" and start feeling pinned up, go for a walk, even if it is only around your back yard. Get out that old treadmill you have buried in the garage set it up and start using it.

Implement a time for working out in your day by turning on an exercise DVD to fight stress before it begins.

Reserve a private area in your home to use as a

peaceful refuge when things get tense. Surround yourself with beautiful plants. This could be your own bedroom or another room in the house that you could set up a stereo with some nature music or soft jazz. Make sure your LO is comfortable and safe and then retreat into a more peaceful surrounding. It can help you regain proper perspective on the anointed calling of caregiving again.

TIP #11:

So, your LO is being stubborn these days about everything. He argues with you about the most ridiculous things. He fights you about taking his medication, taking a bath and accuses you of trying to steal his money. He causes strife between you and your other relatives by lying about your intentions (and they usually believe him!) and all of this makes you very angry.

Remember this; there will come a time when you would give anything to hear his voice again; to see him, regardless of the difficulty of his demands and the trouble he causes.

One day, when he has passed on, you could feel this way, so make the most of the time left.

Try to find the humor in everyday situations and then write them down in a journal. Look back on them when you need to be reminded of his humanity. This can help you to regain your perspective and your self-control.

TIP #12:

After you have been physically or verbally abusive, if you find yourself feeling guilty, apologizing, and then doing it repeatedly, you are a serial abuser. Your personality is changing and it will take its toll on you emotionally, morally and physically if you do not get some help.

Join a support group for family caregivers where there is safe haven for emotions to vent and deal with, without shame.

Make sure to apply Tip # 8 immediately before it is too late and you really hurt your LO.

TIP #13:

The bible clearly says, "Whatsoever you sow, that surely shall you also reap." Reflect on turning contempt into compassion. Make it your new goal to start sowing good seed and spray the weed killer of repentance over the bad crops.

Understand this: If God did not call you to provide care for someone with dementia, family or not, you are not equipped to do so physically, emotionally, mentally or spiritually. You will not have the patience or wisdom required to care for them effectively and that is the least they deserve.

YOU HAVEN'T FAILED!

There are two situations you must adjust to when you take

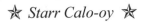

on the care of a full-grown adult; (1) coping with a flood of mixed emotions and (2) the daily hands on care.

If your LO had been diagnosed with a rare and painful type of cancer, and he had to be admitted to a facility that specialized in dealing with the pain, would you feel guilty if your doctor told you he needed to be admitted to a pain management clinic?

Of course not! You would be grateful that there was such a place to help him. There would be no way that you could possibly make a difference in his care or the outcome, no matter how much you loved him or how long you had been together.

If you are honest and admit to yourself that you truly have a problem in this area, then you will perform the most loving and compassionate act for your LO by exploring alternate living arrangements.

This is not about you failing at caregiving- It is not about you at all. It is about your LO receiving the care he deserves in the autumn of his life. If you are not up to it, then do something about it now.

PLAN OF ACTION FOR DEALING WITH ANGER IN YOUR ELDERLY LO!

TIP # 1:

Above all, do not argue or debate with your LO. You cannot possibly win.

You will really want to, especially if you're caring for a parent who always had the last word. If he has always gotten his way and disregarded your opinions and feelings when you were young and too little and helpless to assert yourself, it will be tempting.

You may feel that you have the upper hand and that he is the helpless one now; that it is payback time.

Please understand this- if you are considering going this route, it borders on abuse. Try and bring peace through forgiving your LO.

After all, how much satisfaction can there possibly be in winning an unimportant argument with a mentally challenged and helpless individual anyway?

Your own self image will go in the dunker very quickly if you behave immaturely and lash out at your LO.

Rationalize your acts of patience and kindness by telling yourself that your LO will not remember how brilliantly you debated with him in 5 minutes anyway! That will give you pause.

TIP # 2:

Entice your LO into another room or to go with you outside, if weather permits. If he is wheelchair bound, this can be easy. If he is ambulatory, it may require a little more persuading. Do yourself a favor and smile as you speak softly, make the suggestion and take him gently by the hand if he will allow it. Sometimes a change of scenery is all that is needed to turn his mood around. Many times, he will completely forget he was even angry.

TIP # 3:

Do not laugh at this one until you try it- it really works! Change your clothes and/or hair, then walk back into the room, and say something like "Well, hello! How have you been?" In other words, start over again. The changes will often cause him to forget that his anger was directed toward you.

We used to keep a couple of nurses' smocks on hand and a stethoscope to hang around our necks. Even the most obstinate person will respect "the uniform."

TIP # 4:

As soon as the conversation gets hot, head for the freezer! We keep emergency bowls of ice cream made up for such times. Our motto is "Ice cream makes the world go round." Once you present him with a sweet treat, he will completely forget he was ever upset at all, so make sure you do not remind him! If his passion is candy, pie or whatever it is, keep it close by and serve it right up to alter his mood.

TIP # 5:

Eliminate all noise within his earshot if possible. Noise can bring on catastrophic reactions faster than any other outside stimuli. If you are in the living room, the TV or radio is on very loud, and there are several family members talking, laughing or arguing, it can really set off someone with dementia.

Remember, his brain cannot filter out the overload to the senses as a well-minded person can. He can become confused when he cannot process what is going on. Take him to a quiet room, free from all movement, bright lights and noise and then slowly and quietly sit with him until he is calm.

If he will allow you to, stroke his hair and tell him how much you love him. Speak softly and remember to smile. Speak in no more than 5 word sentences, get at his eye level, and above all, remember to smile. Do not question him.

TIP # 6:

Many angry reactions can be prevented by simply explaining what you are doing before working with your LO.

For example: if he gets angry at bath time, ask yourself if you are jerking him around roughly and not taking time to explain **each step** of the process as you go. Tell him "I am going to help you bathe. Now I am going to take your shirt off. Now let's take off your pants." And "I am going to put water on your hair to wash it."

I have found it useful to make sure they remain covered by a towel as I bathe different parts of their body. This way they still keep their dignity, don't feel molested or give me an argument.

Do not assume that he should know the routine by now and that he does not need any warning as to the steps of the process. He needs to be told each time. His memory is nothing like yours. Treat them as such.

TIP # 7:

Do not rush him. Take your time to move in slow motion. To move at a normal pace can cause a catastrophic reaction.

Again, I cannot say it enough- speak softly and slowly in 5 word or less sentences, using eye contact at his eye level.

TIP # 8:

Do not expect him to do anything if he is tired or not feeling well that day. We do not like to be forced to do even the simplest tasks when we feel bad or tired.

We have a hard time concentrating.

Much more so, for someone who is mentally impaired. They have lost all social awareness and they wear their hearts on their sleeves- they have a lack of self-control and will physically and /or verbally let you know if you are upsetting them. Their emotions are greatly amplified above ours and are extremely sensitive.

TIP # 9:

Do not overload him with instructions. If he has to think of too many things at the same time and remember how to do them, regardless of how easy they seem to you, he can get frustrated and lash out at you as an act of self-defense.

Lead him one step at a time in short sentences, speaking softly and smiling all the while, telling him what you want him to do.

When he completes one step, slowly move to the next and be sure to praise him! Simply stop the activity if you see he is starting to get stressed out- it's just not worth it.

TIP # 10:

How about just leaving him alone? What a novel idea! Give him his space. If you are trying to get him ready to go somewhere or to take a bath, wait 10 minutes and then try it again. OR, you could try having another family member take a shot at it- but again, after at least 10 minutes have passed.

Above all, express your love in words, with touch and facial expressions. Mercy, grace, forgiveness and love are the most effective ways to handle anger and will quench even the most fierce, raging fire within your LO.

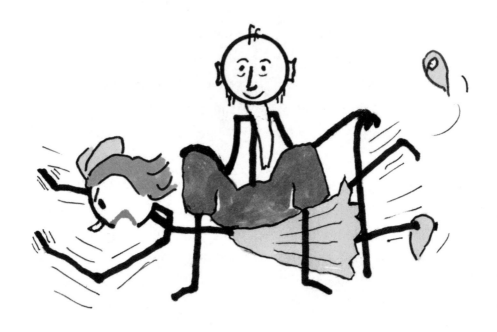

Everybody was
Kung Fu fighting

-B-

BEHAVIORAL PROBLEMS

THIS CHAPTER:

- **Agitation & Combativeness**
- **Paranoia**
- **Rummaging, Pillaging, Hoarding**
- **Wandering**

BEHAVIORAL PROBLEMS

Have you ever found yourself saying, "Who are you and what have you done with my father?" Invasion of the body snatchers?

Sometimes it feels like that, doesn't it? I mean, he looks like your dad, sounds like him but you cannot believe that he could act like that!

You were living in your house, going about your own life and you were at peace with the world and everyone in it when all of a sudden, your LO began acting strange.

You find yourself having to address situations with him, his neighbors, friends and your relatives. Then, your life is taken over with one emergency after another.

You do not know how to reach him anymore. He doesn't seem to be listening or is tuning you out. He is forgetting entire conversations and you wonder if he is doing all of this on purpose, but if so, why?

You also wonder if you'll ever get your life back. You have to make excuse after excuse for canceling your own appointments, time off from work and time with your husband or immediate family.

In this chapter, we will attempt to help you understand what is going on by identifying particular behaviors that are

common in the elderly. Then, we will give you numerous tips on how to help both of you and bring some peace into your lives.

AGITATION & COMBATIVENESS

Imagine, you don't know what's wrong, but you do know that something is just not right. You don't know where you are or who all these people are around you. The noise makes it even harder to try and figure this out. If you only saw someone you knew, you could ask them. You need to go to the bathroom but you don't know where it is. You start to fidget. You discover you are pacing back and forth. You stop one person and then another and then another but no one understands your words. This is a nightmare!

No one knows for sure why someone with dementia gets agitated but it may be that the changes in the brain are more prevalent than other times.

Usually when they are fatigued, the agitation becomes heightened. When they cannot adequately express their needs or feelings, they get anxious.

If your LO has lost something dear to him, he can get very upset and stuck; for the duration of the day, he will obsess over it, even if you put it in his hand.

If others in your home are upset, he will mirror these feelings.

If he is being hurried to do something, like get ready, he can suddenly start crying, get angry or start pacing.

Pain, fatigue, depression, incorrect medication, over-stimulation and restlessness can all be causes of agitation.

Agitation in a well-minded person manifests in a wide variety of ways. For example:

- Impatience
- Anger
- Wandering
- Trying to escape the house
- Intolerance
- Worry
- Nervousness
- Physical or verbal altercations
- Quarreling

However, when someone with AD gets agitated, unusual behaviors that have nothing to do with the situation, become apparent. For example:

- Repetitive questions or comments
- Pacing
- Fidgeting
- Verbal outbursts
- Combativeness

Below, I've listed some ways to help your LO relax.

AGITATION PLAN OF ACTION!

TIP # 1:

Check his diaper to see if it's wet. He could be uncomfortable, unable to verbalize it and you not be aware of it.

TIP # 2:

He may be hungry or thirsty. Offer him a non-sugar, but sweet treat, if it's between meals. Get him some juice and see if he accepts it. Do not give him anything caffeinated.

TIP # 3:

Stay calm and be gentle in your actions and verbiage. Smile and speak slowly. Don't question him repeatedly.

TIP # 4:

Go for a walk with him. If he is wheelchair bound, take him for a stroll if the weather is nice. Some fresh air and a change of scenery is all it takes to calm him sometimes.

TIP # 5:

Give him something safe to fool with, like a pocket of pennies or a strand of beads. Give him something "to do" so he will be distracted from his emotional discomfort.

TIP # 6:

If the doctor has okayed it and it won't interfere with his meds, give him a glass of wine and join him!

TIP # 7:

If you notice that he grows agitated with several people in the same room as he, take him out or ask the others to leave the room.

TIP # 8:

Give him one instruction at a time to cut down on the confusion which leads to agitation. Give him time to respond after an instruction. Remember, his brain needs to sort out the correct response and he is searching much like you sort through a file cabinet for the right file.

TIP # 9:

Choose his best time of day to do something that will require him to follow your lead. After caring for him for a few weeks, you will come to know what his best time is.

TIP # 10:

If he starts to get upset, stop the activity, if possible. Nothing is worth his discomfort.

TIP # 11:

Don't argue, explain or try to reason with him while he is agitated.

TIP # 12:

If you make the mistake of trying to restrain him instead of simply walking away or out of his reach, you'll only make things worse and extend the time of his recovery.

TIP # 13:

If he is accustomed to you touching him lovingly, try that.

TIP # 14:

If he is severely agitated, call his doctor or nurse and ask them for their suggestions. They may prescribe an anti-anxiety medication for him.

PARANOIA

It seems as if your LO has suddenly begun to suspect everyone he meets and believe there is a conspiracy to rob him of everything he holds dear. There is nothing you can say to alleviate him from this mental and emotional distress and you feel hopeless. Sound familiar?

The most common misconceptions that cognitive-impaired people suffer from are listed below:

1. The fear that people, any and all people, are out to steal their money and possessions.
2. The fear that people are out to poison them in their food, drink or medications.
3. The belief that their family and friends are dangerous strangers even to the point of the compulsion to repeatedly call the police.
4. The belief that friends and family who have died are still alive.
5. The fear that everyone is out to kill them, to the point that normal, routine care is difficult.

Some of the reasons for this behavior are:

- They lack the ability to remember. Because they have stashed their valuables in a safe hiding place and now cannot remember exactly where that safe place is, the confusion leads them to believe someone has stolen them.

- The majority of their possessions have been sold or stored so they can move into a facility or someone else's home. They cannot see their things and now nothing looks familiar. Their surroundings that they had grown so accustomed to have changed and they cannot remember why. Things seem to be disappearing all around them and they have no control over their environment. They will panic over even the most insignificant things (to us) when they have seemingly "disappeared."

- We are taught from the earliest age to be cautious about strangers. Now, everyone is a stranger so they remain in a suspicious state. Depending on a person's upbringing, they may have been taught prejudice based on race, religion, "shifty eyes", gender or even by what a person wears. As the dementia deepens, so do these ingrained beliefs and opinions.

- Your LO cannot remember the explanation you just gave

him. Even if you have explained the same thing 50 times you must realize that he cannot retain the information. He is not trying to make you angry or frustrate you on purpose. He cannot help it.

- The dementia makes some people overreact to normal situations. Cognitive impaired people often are hyper-sensitive. They will read danger into many things we take for granted. A new face or place can be terrifying to them. From their mentally twisted viewpoint, all they can see is that nothing happens without a major significance and that anything that happens is related to them. They lack the ability to properly assess what is actually happening so they suspect everyone who comes into their view or hearing and live in constant fear.

PARANOIA PLAN OF ACTION!

TIP #1:

Before you do anything, you must have the proper mindset yourself! Do not take what they are saying or doing personally. This is not about you. It is about the dementia and your LO. It doesn't matter if they were ogres when you were little. The first step is to forgive anything you believe they did to you in the past, even the recent past just before they exhibited signs of dementia.

Many people find it difficult to remember the point at which their LO first began to change. They look back and reflect certain events that occurred and realize the turning point after the fact. Try and remember that your LO is helpless and needs your understanding, compassion, patience and loving kindness now.

TIP # 2:

Be helpful! Offer to look for what is missing even if it doesn't exist. They are in your care and depend on you to make them feel secure. Give them a substitute if you can. Show them that you are their advocate, not their enemy.

TIP # 3:

Try and keep the room your LO is in quiet and operating at a slow pace to avoid confusion as much as is possible. Loud noise will excite and cause them to overreact. All of their senses are heightened so keep this in mind when preparing the atmosphere. It may seem like a lot of work to do this daily but look at the alternative. Wouldn't you rather take a few measures beforehand than have a combative, angry upset elderly LO to try and calm down?

TIP # 4:

Stick to the same routine every day as much as possible. Changes can jar them in to a catastrophic emergency. This means give them their bath at the same time and the same way every time. They should eat at the same table, in the same spot, at the same time every day. It is a proven fact that people with dementia find great solace in routine even though they do not remember what happened 5 minutes ago. You may think that going for a car ride would be nice for them but many times it will upset them greatly and it can take hours for them to readjust after they get back home. The unfamiliar is frightening so protect them from it.

TIP # 5:

If they refer to you or someone else as a departed person or talk about them as if they were still alive, do not correct them and tell them that the person is dead. This might depress your LO or cause them to become angry and it serves no purpose anyway. You aren't there to correct their mindset or teach them anything anyway. Your purpose is to make them feel as safe, secure and at peace as possible is not it? If you have to play along with what they believe to be so then do it and with a smile to boot!

TIP # 6:

Watch their sugar and caffeine intake. Dementia patients have a very delicately balanced system. Sometimes all it takes is a Cup of caffeine-laden coffee to cause them to completely change from their usual sweet self to believing you are a spy in a James Bond movie for the OTHER side.

TIP # 7:

Ask your LO's doctor to

re-evaluate their meds to make sure there is no conflict. Sometimes, paranoia can be the result of a poor combination of a new medication and the old ones.

Ask the pharmacist for a printout on all medications they are taking and see if he will check to see if they are safe if taken together.

You'd be surprised at the side effects of taking certain medications with others.

TIP # 8:

Crowds can be especially devastating to those with dementia. Large rooms filled with people and noise can cause them to feel extremely paranoid and lead to anger and suspicion. Try and avoid taking them out into this type of atmosphere at all cost. Even at home you will find a small quiet room will alleviate many behavioral problems.

Do not ever laugh at them, no matter how comical they are. Their fear, although unfounded and imaginary, is very real to them and they look up to you as their hero; their protector. Do not let them down.

RUMMAGING, PILLAGING & HOARDING (RPH)

Does this sound at all, unpleasantly familiar? "Where on earth did I put my keys? I hung them up last night when I got home, I think? Betty, have you seen my keys? I am late enough as it is. Are you sure you did not move them when you cleaned up last night?"

And then it slowly dawns on you, as this nauseating churning in the pit of your stomach begins.

"Betty! Check your mother's room. Look in her closet behind the red shoes. See if they're in there and hurry!" Sure enough, Betty saves the day and finds her hysterical husband's keys and another mysterious case of the hoarder is solved.

Betty's mother has Alzheimer's disease and tends to take anything that suits her little fancy that is lying around. Nothing is safe. Nothing is sacred.

The person with Alzheimer's does not attach any particular monetary value on the things they take and hide. It could be a bar of used soap, a remote control, assorted shoes, socks or other pieces of clothing that do not fit them. So why do they do it?

No one really knows for sure, but there are a few theories out there and I will share some of mine with you.

They may pick something up, play with it a while and then forget where they got it from a few minutes later, so they just stash it out of sight.

They may be reliving their childhood days; a time when they were very poor and had very little. They exhibit "stockpiling" tendencies because they are fearful that later on they will be without once again and they might have need for the item. This behavior makes them feel secure and that, in a sense, they are providing for the future.

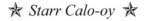

They may feel that they are helping out by cleaning up the clutter around the house.

RPH Plan of Action!

TIP# 1:

Have duplicates of things you need and cannot live without like keys, hearing aide batteries and eyeglasses just in case your LO pillages them.

TIP# 2:

If you do not want your LO to have access to specific drawers or cabinets, then secure them with childproofing hardware or locks.

TIP# 3:

Get rid of the clutter.

TIP# 4:

Look through your wastebaskets before the trash is thrown out.

TIP# 5:

Take note where your LO "stashes" things. They tend to return to the same location each time they retrieve their little trophy.

TIP# 6:

Lock up some of the rooms in the house so that your residing hoarder has fewer places to hide things and you have fewer places to search.

TIP# 7:

Make up their own little trays of fake jewelry, old keys (that do not work anymore!) and trinkets that are safe for them to pick up.

<u>TIP# 8</u>:

Give them small shopping bags and a few old purses to satisfy their compulsion and keep them safely busy while you get your housework done.

THE "DO NOTS"

- **Do not** panic, scream, and cry in front of them.
- **Do not** yank your things out of their hands- offer to "trade" them instead. Most importantly, do not fail to keep your sense of humor. You're going to need it!
- **Do not** leave important things lying around.
- **Do not** keep your money in plain sight.

WANDERING

The family who is caring for a LO with Alzheimer's disease in their own home, has to be ready to deal with a variety of unusual behavioral tendencies. One of these traits is wandering.

There are specific precautions that you can take to avoid your LO from getting lost.

You need to understand that someone with Alzheimer's has the inclinations of a little child. They are easily distracted by anything that catches their eye- bright colors and delightful sounds that will soothe their soul. They will also revert to habits they formed in their younger years such as jobs and chores and may leave your presence in order to fulfill their "obligations".

There may other reasons they wander as well. They may be trying to handle the stress of their environment, which they may view as being noisy, crowded, isolated, or unpleasant. They may go out in search of such basic needs as food, water or a bathroom and have simply lost their way trying to find them. They may be trying to find familiar faces, objects surroundings or companionship. Maybe they have misinterpreted certain sights or sounds as being life threatening or frightening.

Whatever the reason, it is especially frustrating and irritating for caregivers but it can soon become more than that when the AD victim moves into an unsafe or unhealthy area or climate, puts others at risk or invades another person's property.

There are steps, which can be taken to avoid irreversible and dangerous situations.

WANDERING PLAN OF ACTION!

TIP # 1:

Encourage exercise and walking in a safe, secured area.

TIP # 2:

Survey your area for possible hazards such as a pool, busy roadways they could wander out into, tunnels, dense foliage, steep stairways, high balconies, bus stops, the absence of fences or gates and unbolted entryways in your home.

TIP # 3:

Use nightlights, cue signs and familiar objects to help them move around the house safely.

TIP # 4:

Make sure they wear something to identify them each day. For example, a necklace with a plate that tells their address, phone number and name and mental/medical condition. They can have their ID on their shoes, glasses or dentures. Always be aware of what they are wearing each day.

TIP # 5:

Keep a list of your neighbors names and phone numbers and let them know that your LO may wander and to keep an eye out. Ask them to gently lead your LO back home if they see them out alone. Explain to them how to do this without arousing them to combativeness or promoting a catastrophic emergency.

TIP # 6:

If your LO is missing, begin to look for him close by. Call his name, inform the neighbors and ask them to help you look. Call the police and fire departments. When you locate him, approach him with calmness and gentleness. Do not scold him. He was on a mission, remember? Have a nice leisurely walk back home.

TIP # 7:

Invest in a wandering device. There are bedside pads that alert you when your LO has gotten out of bed. A security system can be just as helpful. Ask a security expert what is available or contact your local Alzheimer's Association and ask them for the latest in safety/security measures for the Alzheimer victim.

TIP # 8:

If your LO is unsteady on his feet and you cannot keep them down safely when you are working in your home and moving from room to room, try a bean bag chair. This chair is very difficult to get up from. At night, try placing their mattress on the floor. This way, they do not have far to fall if they try and get up in the middle of the night. They most probably will not be able to get up at all. Make sure you move

anything they could knock over in their relentless efforts to get up and out though. You do not want anything falling on their head and compounding the problem.

TIP # 9:

Ask your physician for a prescription request for a Geri-Chair. This marvelous invention is a chair that reclines with a built in tray which fits nicely over their lap preventing them from getting up- in MOST cases that is. You may find that Houdini doesn't have anything on your LO when it comes to escape tricks!

TIP # 10:

Give your LO something to do like counting pennies, folding clothes or sorting playing cards. Try anything that can use up their energy

and cause them to re-focus
and get their mind off of

trying to get out of the
house.

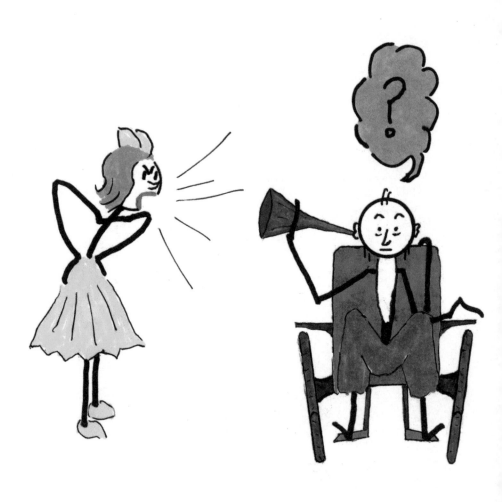

Yakety-Yak

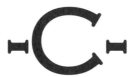

COMMUNICATING EFFECTIVELY

THIS CHAPTER:

- **Ask**
- **Listen**
- **Noise**
- **Distractions**
- **Questions**
- **Redirect**
- **Respect**
- **Smile**
- **Speak slowly**

COMMUNICATING
EFFECTIVELY

One of the most irritating experiences
for a caregiver, friend or family
member to go through, is trying to
effectively communicate to their LO with
dementia.

The reason for the frustration is that we
are coming from a well-minded point of
reference and expecting a similar response.

This is impossible because their world is
filled with confusion and no longer makes
sense. They may understand what is being

said, but may not be able to form the words to respond in intelligible sentences.

They may substitute certain words or phrases in place of what we would to communicate, but to them, it makes sense.

Keep in mind that it is extremely frustrating for them also, when they are in the early stages of dementia. Later on, it does not really matter to them, mercifully so.

As dementia progresses, it becomes increasingly difficult to know how to adhere to their wishes or figure out why they are unhappy or uncomfortable.

There are several ways that you can optimize your chances to understand them. Below are a few tips for you, the caregiver, and visitors to keep in mind while attempting to make contact:

PLAN OF ACTION!

TIP #1:

Remember when you meet, do not expect anything from your LO. People with dementia do not respond the same as well minded people. This means do not expect them to be happy you came to visit because they may not even know who you are now or they may be angry with not only you, but also everyone because of their confusion so do not take it personal. Do not try and analyze why they are talking and acting like they are. You cannot accurately empathize with a person who has dementia, when you are coming from a well-minded perception.

TIP #2:

Do not expect them to ask forgiveness. They probably do not recall all the harsh words and actions between both of you from the past. Do not be offended if they do not remember and think that they just do not care or that they have to be faking memory loss. Remember, they may look close to the same as the last time you saw them, but if they have dementia, they are not. Be prepared to accept their state of mind, whatever it is.

TIP #3:

Do not ask them questions about anything or anybody. Many people make the mistake of starting most sentences with the words, "Do you remember?" Questions will stress them out due to word finding problems and they will have difficulty answering you as well as understanding all that you say. Let them lead and if they ask you questions, answer in sentences of no more than 6 words, and repeat it if necessary, otherwise they may not be able to follow the conversation.

Tip # 4:

Never approach them physically from behind or you may startle them. When you talk to them, make sure that you are physically on their level, directly in front of them, making direct eye contact.

Tip # 5:

Smile at them when you speak. If you do, you will not cause them to feel threatened in any way and your visit has a better chance of being successful.

Tip # 6:

Speak to them in a slow, low and even tone, enunciating each word so that you are sure to be heard and understood.

Tip # 7:

If they are hard of hearing, speak loudly but again, be sure to smile so that they do not misinterpret what you say as your being angry with them.

Tip # 8:

If they are in the stage of dementia where they speak "word salad" (words that do not form sentences when put together), **do** not (and I strongly emphasize this) correct them. Just smile and go along with them. Do not embarrass them or make them feel belittled.

If there have been hard feelings in the past between you, you may have the tendency to use their vulnerability and weakness as an outlet for revenge. You are not there to exact judgment but to give mercy and grace and to vaporize your guilt phantom.

Remember, say yes, each time their voice inflection goes up as in a question addressed to you. This will set their mind at ease even if you do not understand the question they seem to ask you.

TIP # 9:

Loving touches, strokes of tenderness and kisses on the cheek are healing, not only to the receiver, but to the sender as well. Because of extraordinary communication problems they may not be capable of understanding your words but the dementia patient will always understand displays of affection.

You can accomplish this without any words at all. By doing this, you will feel better about your relationship and it will actually put you on the road to recovery in regard to emotionally being unable to visit with them in the past.

If you have shown true forgiveness in the form of a loving touch, kind words and actions, when you get home you will become aware of the absence of the guilt phantom that has stalked you for so long.

TIP # 10:

Don't try to teach your

LO how to communicate with you because it's a waste of time and will only frustrate him. You must learn how to connect with him.

TIP # 11:

Keep in mind that he will mirror your body and facial language as well as your attitude toward him. Keep it light.

TIP # 12:

Keep distractions and noise away from him while attempting to work with him.

TIP # 13:

Speak in 3-5 word sentences. Repeat slowly and watch your tone. Make sure you use low pitch commands.

TIP # 14:

If he gets distracted, redirect him. This will require a great deal of patience on your part.

TIP # 15:

Respect him in the manner you speak to him- don't "baby talk" him. He is an adult with speech and cognitive problems.

TIP # 16:

If he doesn't want to talk or listen, don't force him to. Wait until he is ready.

TIP # 17:

Don't waste your time trying to reason with him. If he says the sky is filled with elephants, let him believe it. You gain nothing by arguing with him or trying to set him straight. Go along with whatever delusions he has as long as they don't make him depressed. If they do, redirect his focus.

TIP # 17:

Don't tell him what to do. Instead, ask him. He should not have to obey you- he is an adult!

TIP # 18:

Don't set your expectations too high on him. Unspoken disappointment manifests itself spiritually. It is not a secret you can keep from him. He will feel it, even through the dementia.

TIP # 19:

Learn to listen for key words he is using so you have a better chance of deducing what he is trying to say to you.

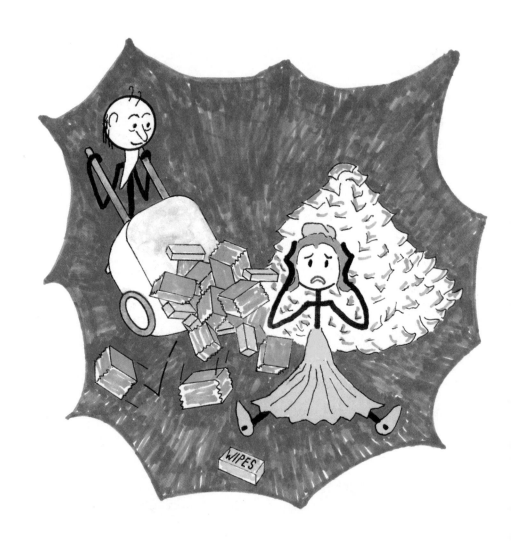

Ain't No Mountain
High Enough

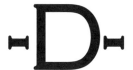

ADULT
DIAPERS

THIS CHAPTER:

- **Changing Adult Diapers**
- **Diaper Rash Tips**
- **How to Keep a Diaper on Your LO**

ADULT DIAPERS

Deterioration of the skin can occur due to uric acid in the diaper area. This can cause painful diaper rash.

If your LO is taking diuretics, such as Furosemide, it will cause them to urinate great volumes daily so be prepared. Unless he wears a bladder catheter, his adult diaper can become full very quickly. If he is not changed regularly, it will eventually cause diaper rash.

Another neat product we use for our high voiding residents is "Diaper Doublers." This amazingly absorbent one-way, thin pad can hold 2 quarts of liquid at a time without spilling a drop! This pad is placed inside the center of the diaper for the male or female. The urine is not only captured, avoiding soiling the outer garments and making it necessary to have to re-bathe your LO, but it keeps the urine away from the skin until you discover you need to change him. Ingenious!

We also recommend moisture barrier ointment that will further protect the skin.

CHANGING AN ADULT DIAPER

(The following is how to clean up a bowel movement, but it is practically the same process if your LO is only wet)

TIP # 1:

You should prepare ahead of time to make your job much easier by remembering to place your LO on a large cloth bed pad with a large paper bed pad on top of it. This way you can throw away most of the loose stools and the cloth pad will catch the remainder and protect the fitted sheet. If you forget once, that'll be all it takes- you <u>will</u> remember next time!

As soon as you discover your LO needs to be changed, get everything ready. You will need:

1. A waste paper container with a new bag
2. A roll of ultra soft paper towels
3. No-Rinse, Peri-wash spray cleanser
4. Baby wipes or warm, moistened paper towels
5. A box of latex gloves
6. Moisture Barrier ointment
7. A new cloth bed pad
8. A new paper bed pad
9. A clean fitted sheet
10. A dirty clothes hamper lined with a plastic bag
11. A diaper
12. Clean clothes (if they have been soiled)
13. Supplies for wound care laid out (if he has bedsores and the dressing has been soiled)

TIP # 2:

The easiest way to get

your LO on the pads without breaking your back, is to:

- First lay the pads (one on top of the other) on top of your LO's body, in the precise position and location you want them to be.
- Then roll them up toward you, but leave the rolls on the bed. They should be lying in one neat roll at his side and on the bed. Do not pick them up.
- Gently roll your LO over on his side facing away from you. Carefully,

unroll the pad roll toward his side until the remainder of the roll meets his back.

- Push the pad set (still rolled up) underneath the side he is laying on and then gently roll him back onto his back.
- Now, reach over him, pull the pads out from under him, and flatten them.
- Roll him onto his back. If you have done it correctly (practice makes perfect!), the pads will be positioned in the right place.

NOW YOU ARE READY TO BEGIN!

- First, wash your hands and dry them well. Put on three pairs of gloves; one on top of another. This way, you can just pull them off and discard as they get dirty. It is very difficult and messy to have to stop in the middle of this procedure to have to put a fresh pair on.

- Remove all loose bedding such as top sheets, blankets and pillows. Allow only one pillow to remain under his head to keep him comfortable.

- If he is lying in a hospital bed, lower the head and knees and raise the bed to a comfortable level so you do not strain your back.

- Breathe through your mouth instead of your nose if you have a weak constitution.

- Undo the tabs on his diaper. Roll him gently away from you onto his side. Pull the diaper down and clean as much of the feces as possible with the inside of the diaper and then roll the soiled part of the diaper into itself and tuck it under his bottom as far as you can.

- Clean him with slightly moistened paper towels first and then with the baby wipes. Place a new bed pad set under the rolled up diaper as far as you can get it.

- With the rolled up soiled diaper under his bottom, go over to the opposite side of the bed and roll him completely over away from you again. Do not forget to pull the bed rail up before you leave one side of the bed to go to the other side, unless, someone is helping you. Pull the new bed pads set out and flatten it so that he now rests on it.

- Repeat the same cleaning procedure for this side and then pull the diaper and soiled paper bed pad out from under him when you are through and throw it away.

- Roll him onto his back, gently open his legs (first, tell him what you are going to do) and clean his front, all creases, and privates.

- Roll him side to side and place the new diaper on him, applying the moisture barrier ointment as you go. If he needs wound care administered, do this after you have cleaned him up and he is on top of his fresh diaper so you do not disturb the dressing.

- If you need to also change the fitted sheet due to soiling, the time to do this is when you are rolling the soiled diaper under him the first time. You can also place the clean fitted sheet on the bed, one side at a time in the process.

- If your LO is a male, be sure to always pull the foreskin on his penis back gently and clean the area well. If you neglect to do this, it will become infected.

- This will take practice, but in time, it will become second nature to you and before you know it, you'll become a pro.

Diaper Rash-Great Tips!

Tip # 1:

Do not use baby wipes. They usually irritate skin with a rash.

Tip # 2:

Do use warm, moist, soft paper towels to clean the area. Wet them, squeeze and shake them out until they open up again.

TIP # 3:

Do not use soap! It is very difficult to adequately rinse soap off the skin and if you aren't successful doing so, it will cause the diaper area to itch and burn causing him to scratch which will cause other problems. Use a no-rinse, spray on cleanser instead. You can pick this up at your pharmacy or a medical supply store.

TIP # 4:

At least 3 times daily, leave his diaper off completely so his skin can air and heal. When you do this, have him lie down but leave the moisture barrier off so the air can get to it.

You can cover him with a light, cotton bed sheet to protect his privacy.

TIP # 5:

Place several paper bed pads underneath him to "catch" the urine or fecal matter but be sure to check him every hour. Replace the wet or soiled bed pads with dry ones as soon as you discover them and then clean his skin immediately.

TIP # 6:

Restrict citrus and carbonated beverages such as juice and sodas until he is clear again. Push the water intake to flush and dilute the uric acid from his system.

Use common sense. If you feel it is more than a common rash, call his doctor to get advice.

Also, in most cases, when your LO is not eating but

drinking liquid supplements and water, he will have very loose bowels. Large bowel movements can be horrifyingly perplexing if you have never had to clean up an adult before. You just do not know where to begin!

Every caregiver has his or her own methodology. With a little practice, you will discover yours.

HOW TO KEEP A
DIAPER ON YOUR LO

It can be messy and frustrating for their loved one to tear up his diaper. Most people would think that the reason their LO takes it off is that he is wet and uncomfortable. Not so. They take off dry diapers as often as wet ones.

Here is the solution. Go to a sporting goods store in your city and purchase a one-piece mechanic outfit that zips up the front. Take the collar off and make a v-neck cut in the back of it and sew it down around the edges. Put it on your LO backwards and zip it up. Now, he isn't able to get to his diaper to take it off anymore.

Just make sure that you check his diaper often so he doesn't get diaper rash.

This same method is useful if your LO is obsessed with going to the bathroom. You know if he's obsessed. He wants to go every five minutes and when you take him, he doesn't urinate the vast majority of the time. Stop taking him every time he asks. Instead, tell him that he is wearing a pad. This is what I usually say in this case:

He says, "I have to go to the bathroom now!" I say, "Go ahead and use your pad right now. I will change it when it's wet. Don't worry- you won't get your pants wet. Someone is in the bathroom right now so we can't go in."

After a couple of days, he will get used to not going to the bathroom, IF you stick to your guns.

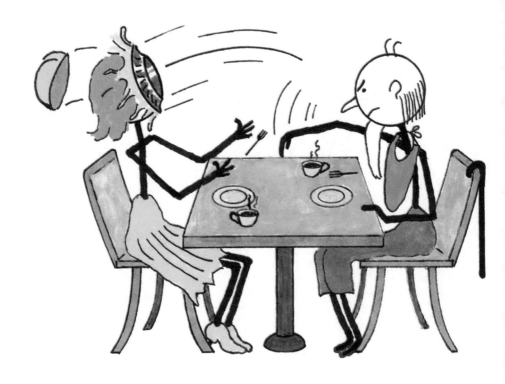

He Ain't Heavy

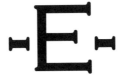

EATING

THIS CHAPTER:

- **The Appestat**
- **Finger Foods**
- **Malnutrition & Dehydration**
- **When He Won't Eat**

EATING

The ritual of eating is one of the most psychologically satisfying activities in which we participate on a daily basis. From the time we are conceived in our mother's womb, we are obsessed about putting something in our mouths.

We associate good times, family gatherings, love, laughter and comfort with food. Food is fuel to our bodies, so when we stop eating, our energy levels go down and if we go long enough, we are no longer resistant to illnesses.

As a caregiver, you must possess a certain amount of creativity when it comes to encouraging your LO to eat. In this chapter, we hope to help you with some productive eating tips.

THE APPESTAT

In order to fully understand why the eating habits of the elderly change as they get older, you need to know about the appestat.

According to Dr. James J. Mahoney D.O. (Founder of The Center for Hope and Healing), *"The appestat is the regulator of hunger and satiety (satisfaction with food). The normal sensation of hunger comes from the body's need for fuel. The stomach is empty, the insulin level has been baseline for some time and the system is beginning to dip into fat reserves for fuel. The feeling of satisfaction or fulfillment comes from the brain's satiety center. This has less to do with hormones and chemistry than it does with the perception and appreciation of food. This is the reason that the most desirable foods MUST be eaten. Without this simple requirement being met, you will stay hungry most of the time no matter what other things you do.*

The hormonal system works to provide a precise signal when the body needs more fuel. Most of us have damaged the sensitivity of our hunger system to the point that it needs rehabilitation. This occurs through several mechanisms. By reducing the stress associated with sugar consumption the remainder of steps seem easy by comparison. Tediously slow chewing reprograms the neurological system of the temperomandibular joint (TMJ). Resting to evaluate stomach fullness resets the neurological systems of stomach feedback. Highest choice food selection reprograms the vital satiety center so that satisfaction is reached early in the feeding process.

You have been programmed to eat more because "it is late" and to drink milk because "it does a body good." I invite you to step up to the controls and do some programming of your own. Eat food you love because you love it. Chew slowly to savor every delicious morsel of your favorite foods. Stop eating when you are comfortable. Enjoy the freedom of eating what you really want while working towards true satisfaction and freedom." Dr. James J. Mahoney

FINGER FOODS

If your LO has difficulty maneuvering eating utensils, try serving finger foods. This may be one reason he has cut down on eating; embarrassment. Be sure to watch the temperature of the food so he doesn't burn his fingers! Listed below are a few suggestions but feel free to be creative and explore your recipe books for more.

- Bacon
- Boiled eggs
- Burritos
- Cheese sticks
- Chicken nuggets
- Chips & dip
- Cookies
- Corn dogs
- Crackers
- Dunken French toast sticks
- Egg rolls
- Fish sticks w/tarter sauce to dip
- French fries
- Fruit
- Granola bars
- Hamburgers

- Hot Pockets
- Hotdogs
- Muffins, rolls, bread sticks, biscuits
- Onion rings
- Quesadillas
- Raw veggies w/dressing to dip
- Sandwiches
- Sausage
- Steak fingers w/gravy to dip
- Tamales
- Taquitos w/guacamole to dip
- Tiny quiches
- Vienna sausage
- Waffles w/syrup to dip

MALNUTRITION & DEHYDRATION

Love will keep us alive. Ah, if this were only so. Unfortunately, if your LO is terminally ill, his appetite will come and go. The very foods he loved all of his life can suddenly hold no special meaning whatsoever. On the other hand, he may begin to request foods he wouldn't touch before.

Illnesses can radically affect our taste for foods. Certain medications have side effects that decrease the appetite.

There will come a time when you cannot get your LO to eat anything. At first, he may ask for a particular meal. Then when you bring it to him, he says he is not hungry or he did not ask for that.

It can be extremely disturbing to a family caregiver for her LO to refuse food or liquids and then witness him waste away right before her eyes.

PLAN OF ACTION!

TIP # 1:

If you begin to see a pattern developing here, try preparing the food once and then if he doesn't eat it, giving him a high caloric liquid supplement like Nestles 2.0 which contains 550 calories per can.

Make a shake with it using his favorite flavored syrup and ice. Tell him he doesn't have to eat that meal if he will drink his shake. Most of the time, I get them to drink every drop when I put it that way. This way, he still gets his nourishment.

TIP # 2:

If you want your LO to drink more fluids and he gets stubborn, tell him if he doesn't drink the water, he will get constipated! This is a true statement and as paranoid as the elderly get about their bowel movements, believe me, he will drink whatever you put in front of him.

As Bob has always said, "The trick is not getting people to do what you want them to do. It is getting them to WANT to do what you want them to do." You have to do whatever it takes to help your LO so he doesn't get dehydrated or starve himself to death.

When your LO nears death, he will reject all substances. This is called "failure to thrive" and the body begins to shut down. If your LO is in this final stage and you force food or liquids in him and they go into his lungs, he can develop pneumonia.

At this point, all organs stop working one by one in preparation for death so you must not fight it. It will not do anyone any good and can cause your LO to drown in the very fluids you are forcing on him.

I know this may sound harsh, but it is a fact and we have had to explain this to many, many families over the past 18 years. Before you make this decision, confer with your family and you LO's doctor.

WHEN HE WON'T EAT

There can be many reasons your LO is not eating. When a baby cries, we usually check his diaper to see if it's wet and remind ourselves of the last time he ate. If these things have been attended to and he still cries after being held, loved and rocked, then by process of elimination, we know to look deeper.

A baby cannot tell you why he is uncomfortable to the point of crying. Many times, your elderly LO will not be able to pinpoint the reason he isn't hungry, so it's up to you to begin your own investigation. Check out some of these reasons/solutions to see if they ring a bell:

1. It could be that his teeth are giving him problems. When was the last time he went to the dentist? You might want to make an appointment for him.

2. If he wears dentures, are they secure? He might not tell you that he has some sore spots underneath. A dentist will be able to tell you if his gums are shrinking. Anyone would lose their appetite if they were in pain.

3. As we age, our sense of taste and smell diminish. Experiment with herbs and spices to learn which ones are more appealing to him. Spicy foods can cause bowel problems, so make sure and be his "pre-taster."

4. Try serving smaller portions. Normal sized portions may be too intimidating and he might not want to hurt your feelings by leaving food on his plate.

5. Make sure the food you serve isn't too well done or crispy because he may have difficulty chewing or swallowing it. Softer food may prove to be a winner. Talk it over with him. Discover his preferences.

6. Some people like things toasted; others like them just warmed. Some like their liquids soupy in food; others like them thick. Ask.

7. If you find that he takes longer to eat at the dinner table, privately discuss everyone's eating slower so he won't feel hopeless or pressured.

PLAN OF ACTION!

TIP # 1:

"Let's make a weekly menu together!" Reminisce with him about the great homemade cooking you grew up enjoying; your favorite breakfasts or dinners and the special meals he was known in the family for preparing.

TIP # 2:

"Let's go grocery shopping!" Ask him to help you make out your grocery lists and then take him to the store with you. Try this for a few weeks and see if it helps to stimulate his appetite. Have him add to the list his favorite foods/brands.

TIP # 3:

"Let's cook together!" Ask him to help you cook or you offer to be his assistant. His interest in food may begin to resurface, as old memories become new ones.

TIP # 4:

We are all going different directions these days and hardly ever eat a meal together as a family. It wasn't always this way. You can probably remember when you were young and your parents called you to all eat at the dinner table together. If you simply prepare his food and sit him down in front of it, the void of the fellowship while eating may cause his appetite to wane. It may be difficult to get all members of the family together at once, but maybe you could all take turns eating with him. Maybe you could take Mondays & Thursdays, your spouse could take Wednesdays & Thursdays and the kids could divide the other days. It's really worth the effort!

TIP # 5:

If he is in good enough health, take him out to eat once a week at his favorite restaurant. Make it a family affair, but be sure to make him the center of attention.

If he cannot get out, bring it home to him and then sit down to enjoy it with him.

When I was caring for my mother in our home, she refused all food until I brought home fried oysters from her favorite restaurant. She was delighted and ate 3 or 4 at a time until they were all gone.

TIP # 6:

If all else fails, order a

liquid nutritional supplement such as Carnation Instant Breakfast, 560 calories per can. It's not only highest in calories, it's chocked full of vitamins and it's delicious. Serve chilled between meals.

TIP # 7:

Check with his doctor or pharmacist to see if one of the side effects of his medication is a loss of appetite. If so, ask your doctor for an alternative medication.

TIP # 8:

If he is depressed (another sign of appetite loss), ask his doctor for an anti-depressant.

TIP # 9:

Keep dry, nutritional snacks out to encourage

him. Nuts, crackers, cookies, pretzels etc. placed in small bowls all around the house might be enticing as hunger strikes. Keep a bowl of fresh fruit out and encourage him to take of it freely. Eat some with him.

TIP # 10:

Keep noise and other distractions to a minimum. Have some quiet, relaxing music on low to make things calm and more pleasant.

TIP # 11:

If he makes a mess while trying to eat, ignore it; don't embarrass him by drawing attention to it by trying to clean him up. Use a long bib (plastic backed) to catch spills.

TIP # 12:

Don't serve too many different dishes at the same meal. Keep mealtime very simple.

TIP # 13:

Serve him 5-6 light meals day rather than 3 normal sized meals.

TIP # 14:

If the food needs cutting, cut it up in the kitchen, before you serve it to him so he doesn't get embarrassed. Preserve his dignity while you perform every act of service for him. This is the ultimate act of love.

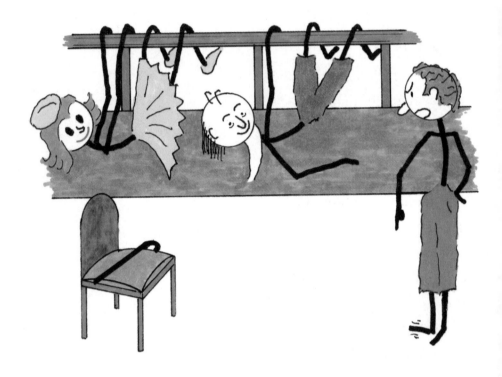

Upside Down

-F-

FAMILY

THIS CHAPTER:

- **Caregiving and Your Marriage**
- **Caregiving and Your Siblings**
- **The Family Gathering**
- **Caregiving and Your Children**

Starr Calo-oy

FAMILY

In the process of caring for the elderly in our home, we have interviewed many weary family caregivers.

They had burned out emotionally, physically and mentally because no one taught them how to take care of themselves. It didn't even enter their minds that they needed care and guidance too. The only thing that mattered to them, was that their LO had dire needs to be met and they were the only ones available to meet them.

When many of them came to us, their marriages were in trouble due to the many demands that the care of their LO made on their personal life.

Their young children were becoming withdrawn emotionally and their teenagers were running wild with little or no regard for parental authority.

Their careers were in shambles, if they still had one. They had used up most or all of their vacation time and sick leave due to trying to juggle the "emergencies" their LO had day after day.

Then, to top it all off, they were running the risk of losing lifelong relationships they had built with their siblings because of conflicting opinions on their parents care..

We helped most of them get their lives back on track through prayer, counseling and leading them through forgiveness.

If you can identify with any of the above, we hope to help you get back on track and stay there to care for your LO with the information in this book.

CAREGIVING AND YOUR MARRIAGE

You had it all planned out. After the children had left the nest, you and your spouse would spend time traveling the world on the savings you had accumulated throughout the years. Great plan, right?

Then it happened, your parent got sick and had to move in with you-permanently.

Now your days are filled with diapers, baths and constant, non-sensical arguments instead of long luxurious cruises. Your nights are spent holding your parents' hand instead of your spouse on warm, sandy beaches. Where did the romance go?

There are some suggestions we want to make to give you back your dreams.

ROMANTIC GETAWAYS

1. Make a list, with your spouse, of all the places you planned to travel before your LO moved in with you. Next to each place on the list, write down the number of days you had planned to be away from home.

2. For your first few trips, select the least number of days to be gone. Put them in order of your preference.

3. PLAN A-----Call your relatives and ask if they would be willing to come and stay at your home so you can go away with your spouse for a few days. When you find a willing sitter, tell her that you will teach her everything she needs to know to care for him. Tell her the date you plan to leave and if this doesn't agree with her schedule, give her an alternate date. Ask her when she can come, then plan your get-away around her plans.

4. PLAN B-----If you can't find a family member to help, try calling a sitters agency from the phone book or ask your LO's doctor for a referral. Then call your family members and ask them to pitch in equally to pay for it. They need to know what it costs you to get away. They take it for granted because they can get up and go anytime they want to.

5. PLAN C----If they aren't willing to help you sit with their LO or pay for someone else to do it, write a check to the sitter from his account that you sign on for you and your spouse to get away. If you have financial (durable) power of attorney for him, this will not be a problem. If you are not, you should be if you are the

primary caregiver. Keep in mind that the money is in his account for his care now. He will not be going home and you aren't taking anyone's inheritance. Inheritance is what's left over after a person has used their money on themselves and that includes their care. If family members aren't willing to care for them, part of their own inheritance will do the job just fine!

TORN: YOUR MARRIAGE VS. YOUR LOVED ONE

Granted, it's very exciting to you now that you finally have your LO at home with you where he will be safe and you can spend more time with him. Make sure you exclude the rest of your family while you make plans for you and your LO.

Before he moves in, have a heart-to-heart with your spouse, not after he is already there. (If he is already in your home when you read this, we have some ideas for you, which follow this section.)

If your LO has trouble sleeping, eating, dressing, bathing etc. discuss the need for your attention with your spouse. Explain to him that this will take time away from him and your children. I'll tell you what- let me tell him- have him read this:

Your spouse is in a very difficult position right now. She knows her dad needs to move in with your family but doesn't want to impose on you or inconvenience you. Her marriage is so important to her but she feels like she has been backed into a corner with no way out. She desperately needs your understanding and compassion. She needs you to handle things as if your own parent needed to move in with the two of you.

This won't last forever, even though at times it may seem like that. This is another season of your marriage that both of you must endure together, as the strong team God made you to be. This is going to mean you must sacrifice time with her and pitch in to help when she asks you to and to do it without complaining. She will never forget the loving ways you put up with her parent and will be ready to give back what you have sown when it comes time to help your parents. She cannot do it alone and she shouldn't have to. She has a great helpmeet in you. Don't let her down now that you both have gone through so much together.

WHEN PARENTS ON BOTH SIDES ARE ILL

There are several ways to handle things when parents on both sides need care.

- Have a family gathering for each family LO needing care. Delegate accordingly.
- If there isn't enough family members able to help out and your LO can still stay at his own home, pay for a live-in aide out of his account to stay with him.
- If there aren't enough family members able to help out and your LO *can't* stay in his own home, pay for a live-in aide out of his account to stay at the primary caregivers home.
- If you cannot find a good live-in, try to hire an aide to come and go each day or two girls who split up the week.

WHEN YOUR LOVED ONE BECOMES VIOLENT WITH YOUR SPOUSE

Usually, the reason an elderly loved one becomes violent is that they have some sort of dementia.

If this is the case, ask you LO's doctor to explain his violent behavior.

If the violence is recurring and only towards your spouse, it may because you look a lot like his spouse when he/she was young and your LO may be exhibiting jealousy. If this is what's happening, make sure that your spouse doesn't show affection toward you in his presence.

Your spouse may resemble someone your LO detested in his younger years. If so, your spouse needs to find things to do to help you out of your LO's sight.

It does absolutely no good to argue verbally with your LO or to try and put shame on him if he has dementia. If he does not have dementia, he may still be jealous of the time you need to spend with the rest of your family. Put your foot down, softly, and stand your ground. They need your attention too. If your LO is fed, loved, dry and comfortable, tell him you need to tend to the rest of the family and then do it. Don't allow him to put shame on you either!

HAPPILY EVER AFTER!

Sometimes you have to be reminded to do things that you do on your own normally. Confused? Well, you won't be after reading the following list.

- Get plenty of rest on the day you plan to have sexual relations with your spouse. Have sex often - it will rejuvenate both of you. You owe it to him and to yourself as well.
- Even in the height of the caregiving experience, smell your sweet best. Bathe regularly. Brush your teeth at least twice a day and use mouthwash. Use your spouse's favorite perfume.

- Keep your hair looking nice and neat.
- Make a list of special things to do for your spouse that you know he really loves. Do one a day. Keep replenishing the list.
- Buy him a thank you card and write down how much his consideration has meant to you.
- Make your spouse his favorite dish and serve it beautifully to him.
- Wake him up with breakfast in bed on a bed tray.
  The point I am trying to make is to make your spouse feel special because he is. Don't let the fire go out of your marriage when your LO comes to stay with you. You need more fire to make it through the hurdles that will come your way now.

CAREGIVING AND
YOUR SIBLINGS

It seems like everyone in the family has an opinion about how you should be taking care of your loved one. However, you are the one family member who stepped up to the plate and moved your parent in with you. You have sacrificed so much and feel that no one really appreciates you.

In fact, all of those old feelings of rivalry and jealousy between you and your siblings came flooding back in, soon after this journey in caregiving began. You didn't sign up for all of this conflict. You have other things more important to be concerned about, like caring for your LO. Why don't they just mind their own business and leave you alone! They just aren't being fair.

Or, maybe you have never been closer to your brothers and/or sisters since your loved one has become sick. For some families, it strengthens the members and for others, it can bring emotions such as resentments and sibling rivalry to the surface they thought was buried long ago.

Does any of this ring a bell? You aren't alone. The vast majority of family caregivers are going through the same thing every day. Actually, family caregiving will change all of your relationships in one way or another. Keep in mind that your various family members do not feel or react the same way as you do. They all have different priorities, opinions, desires, beliefs and backgrounds.

Just of a few of the factors that mold people in different ways are:

- growing up and living in contrasting homes
- health changes
- unique lifestyles
- job/career alterations
- family additions
- growth in diverse places
- losses and gains in distinct areas

Regardless of how well you knew your brothers or sisters while you were growing up, if you haven't lived with them the majority of the past year, you do not know them. Don't expect too much from them. Have empathy for what you know about your family. Have compassion and consideration for what you may not know; this may be causing them to act in unbecoming ways. Be long-suffering and show loving-kindness. People handle emotional pain and disappointment in many different ways.

Whatever you do, don't become self-righteous, legalistic or judgmental. Adult males seem to have much more difficulty handling their emotions when it comes to seeing their parents frail and helpless. Many of them can't bring themselves to visit or help with the hands-on care. This doesn't necessarily mean that you love your parents more than they do or that they are taking advantage of you. There are plenty of jobs they can help you with which will require phoning, legwork and other time-consuming tasks you don't have time to do while you are caregiving.

You may be tempted to feel that they don't understand you have a life too- that they must think their life has more demands on their time than yours does. However, if you are as wise as a serpent and gentle as a dove, you will be able to elicit all the help you need. First, we need to get organized.

THE FAMILY GATHERING

Call all of your siblings and ask them to attend a family meeting at your home or at one of their homes. Whichever is more convenient for all concerned.

Tell them that the reason for your meeting is for each of you to bring a list of your concerns regarding the future plans regarding your parent. This can include:

1. Your parents' financial state
2. A report on your parents state of health
3. Living arrangements for you parent
4. Transportation to and from doctor appointments
5. Cooking
6. Cleaning
7. Laundry

What I suggest is a bit unconventional, but it can work. Let's say that the majority of the family says they don't have time to do the primary caregiving. They don't want to give baths or anything that directly has to do with hands-on care. Fine. This is the case in most families.

Don't force these issues- there is more than enough work to go around. Delegate the work- here is what's up for grabs:

THE VOLUNTEER LIST

- Cooking- This person agrees to cook for your entire family so you can tend to your loved ones personal needs. They can bring the prepared food over weekly or bi-weekly. This would be their ONLY responsibility.

- Cleaning- This person comes over a minimum of 3 times a week to do a thorough cleaning of the house and take out the trash. This would be their ONLY responsibility.
- Laundry- This person comes over to do laundry 4 times a week- to wash, fold, put & hang up all laundry. This would be their ONLY responsibility.
- Appointments & Transportation- This person would handle all appointments and transportation for your LO. He would write all of them on your calendar to keep you up to speed. He would also get him ready for these appointments.
- Yard work- This person would keep your yard looking great- mowing and edging once a week.

Now, be prepared ahead of time for your dependable family members to sweetly ask you what do *YOU* plan to be doing while they do all this work. Sweetly smile. Take a deeeep breath and say:

"To begin with, I have moved dad in to our home and he now occupies one of our bedrooms. Our entire lifestyle has changed. This has affected every member of our family. While all of you are sleeping peacefully through the night, I am up with him because he can't sleep all night. He wants to talk, eat or even go for a walk- at 3 in the morning! I still have to get up at 6 to get ready to go to work.

I change his diapers and clean his genitals. I bathe him amidst his loud protests and angry outbursts. I dress and

undress him at least 3 times a day. I make sure he eats healthily; planning his menus, encouraging him with every bite and occasionally getting food flung in my face. I clean up his messes every day. I plan his activities and participate in them because I am his primary playmate. I shave him, keep his nails trimmed and clean, keep his teeth brushed and make sure he gets enough exercise so his legs don't get stiff. I watch out for all health problems by paying close attention to every part of his body every day of his life.

I do all of this plus hold down a full time job outside the home. This is the reason I am insisting on all of you pitching in to help me take care of this person we all love. Do any of you have a problem with that? Now, who wants to do what on this list?"

If they don't want to do this, suggest they all pitch in $50.00-$75.00 each week to get a maid. Leave it up to them. Just make it clear that you can't do it all by yourself and you shouldn't have to.

If they don't want to pitch in the money or help with the work, announce that you are going to hire a maid to do their jobs and pay them out of dad's account.

Make sure that you have invited aunts, uncles, and cousins etc. to attend this gathering. You will need a lot of help. Don't be disappointed when those you thought would be the first to volunteer, get very quiet and step back to let others take on the more difficult work. In fact, don't be disappointed about anything.

CAREGIVING AND YOUR CHILDREN

Okee-dokee. If you still have children living at home when your LO moves in with you, you are going to have to have a heart-to-heart talk with them. The following is a sample list of items to address, but add to or subtract from them, as you feel led.

- Discuss the reasons why your LO cannot live by himself anymore.
- Tell them why he must live with you instead of any of the other relatives.
- Tell them the room you and your spouse have decided for him to stay in.
- Give them an idea of his physical/mental state.
- If he has dementia, start teaching classes to them and your spouse. Now is a good time to learn about it.
- Tell them what their role will be in helping out. Explain sacrifice, duty, loyalty and basic humanity to them. Tell them life isn't fair. Teach them about sowing and reaping.
- Tell them you really need their help now than ever before and that Granddaddy won't be around forever. Someday, they will really miss him. Now they can get to know him so they can tell their children about him.
- Ask them to share their comments and feelings.
- Tell them that you and your spouse will have a weekly

meeting to discuss complaints and take suggestions to making things run smoother in the house. Then, be sure you do it!

If you find that your children are acting out in school or at home, be patient and allow them to talk to you- you listen. Their response to elder illness is different than an adult's response.

Whatever you do, drop everything if you sense they want to talk to you. These opportunities are rare, so nurture them when they come.

Share your own feelings about your LO and what has happened. Be honest. It can compel them to open up more widely to you.

If your children refuse to help at first, allow it. Don't force them. This situation has already taken their mother's attention away from them, changed the atmosphere in the home and the living quarters may have become strained. Allow them to become emotionally acclimated to your LO and the new set of circumstances without shame and blame.

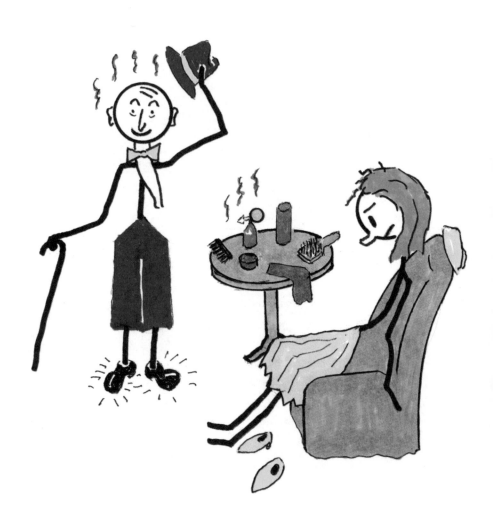

He's So Fine

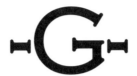

GROOMING

THIS CHAPTER:

- **Bathing**
- **Hair care**
- **Shaving**
- **Oral care**
- **Nail care**

GROOMING

Are you ready for another paradigm shift? Well, here goes! Let's try a little logic. The fact that your LO is now living with you says that he cannot care for himself, right?

Even if he is fully ambulatory and appears to know what he is doing most of the time, he still needs care 24/7 or he wouldn't have had to move in with you. It is up to you now to make sure he is clean and well groomed.

Grooming is a significant part of care. I remember the first time my mother asked me to come to the bathroom with her (at her house). After all of the patients I cared for so many years, it still felt awkward.

She made it easy for me because she needed the help so desperately, that embarrassment was a mute point. This lessened my own embarrassment considerably. That day, it dawned on me that the time of caring for her on a full time basis was approaching fast.

BATHING

At first, it can be rather uncomfortable, not to mention embarrassing, to have to touch your parent's genital area to clean it, but it has to be done.

Keep in mind that there is no one else to do it and put yourself in his place; what if it were you lying in that bed, helpless, weak, with dementia and without the ability to clean yourself? You would want someone to care about your body as you would. We are not saying it is easy but it is necessary. The fact that you are opting to care for him at home while he is dying is the greatest act of love you could ever perform.

We have spoken to many families who have had monumental problems with getting their LO to bathe or to even allow someone else to bathe them.

People with dementia who are combative seem to be more of a challenge, but even the non-verbal and gentle-natured elderly can turn irate and physical when bath time arrives.

There are diverse opinions among the medical professionals as to the reasons for the aversion to bathing. I'll share our opinions, experiences and solutions with you and hopefully you will find a tip or two that will make life easier for both of you.

SOUNDS

Keep in mind that sights and sounds can be amplified many times over with those who exhibit dementia. The mere sound of running water may be extremely frightening to him. It could sound like an avalanche about to fall on his head.

Because of the strain, the time factor and the unpleasantness, most family members elect to give their LO a bath only 2-3 times weekly.

Any non-routine activity you ask your LO to participate in can, in their own mind, present danger and a threat to his safety. If he is exposed to these unfamiliar sounds so rarely it can cause a catastrophic reaction such as violent or abusive outbursts.

SIGHTS

Most bathrooms come equipped with a mirror. Mirrors can cause a person with dementia great confusion. You must remember that things you take for granted every day loom large and scary to your LO. Your reflection as his caregiver can make him believe there are two of you. To avoid this, keep his back towards the mirror or cover it.

Also, he may believe that a naked person is occupying the same small room as himself and when you proceed to disrobe him he can become alarmed.

He may already have word finding problems or difficulty communicating at all, so all he knows to do is to physically defend himself and may, at times, strike out as best he can to fend off the imagined aggressor.

COMMUNICATION TIPS FOR BATHING AN ADULT IN THE SHOWER/TUB

The following are some actions that can cause and prevent your LOs and reluctance and fear of bathing:

PLAN OF ACTION!

TIP # 1:

Do not rush him. Be patient, take your time and do not start a bath unless you have plenty of time to complete it cheerfully.

TIP # 2:

Keep yourself from talking loudly if he is not

hard of hearing. Instead, speak softly and in very short sentences and whenever possible, look into his eyes while speaking and always remember to smile. If he does have hearing difficulties, speak a little louder but make sure you do not frown.

TIP # 3:

Do not pull at his clothes or yank him around – Rather, ask him to help you. For example: When you enter the bathroom, start with a familiar activity like going to the toilet. When you have taken his pants down and he is seated on the toilet, take the opportunity to slip off his shoes, socks and pants. He

may object, so say, "I'm going to help you take your bath." He may reply "I do not need/want a bath. I just took one last night." (Even if he did not).

TIP # 4:

Whatever you do, DO NOT start a debate. You not only will not win, but you'll turn a 30 minute bath into 4 hours trying to win! Stay in motion. You aren't asking his permission, just addressing his concern. Gently proceed disrobing him and talk about his childhood or some subject that is meaningful to him. Anything to distract him from the unpleasantness of "the dreaded bath"!

PLAN OF ACTION!
PRACTICAL TIPS-HOW TO BATHE AN ADULT

TIP # 1:

Try and keep his usual routine as much as possible. Bath time should be planned at the same time and on the same days each week. This way, you will have the least resistance.

TIP # 2:

Before you take him to the bathroom, have the bath water ready, or if you are giving him a shower, the water set at the correct temperature. Have all bath supplies (liquid pump soap, washcloth, towels, shampoo, toothbrush with the toothpaste already on it, floor mat, powder and lotion) laid out to make the ritual as easy as possible.

TIP # 3:

As a distraction technique, have a safe object at hand for him to "play" with while you tend to him. This will make it much easier for you to perform the care and keep him calm.

TIP # 4:

Never leave him alone in the bathtub. He could change the temperature of the water and burn himself.

TIP # 5:

If your LO is very confused and resistant, consider wearing a white nurses uniform. The elderly respect a uniform and the authority that comes with it. As far as he is concerned, you are a doctor or a nurse and have the right to direct him.

TIP # 6:

Use a shower bench whether you are giving him a bath or a shower. It can be extremely difficult for both of you to have to get him up and down to the bottom of a tub, especially when he is wet and slippery.

TIP # 7:

Use a minimum amount of soap to make the rinsing easier. Avoid using oils in the tub area altogether.

TIP # 8:

If he is overweight, make sure you clean any flaps or folds of skin and rinse them well to avoid a rash. When it is time to dry them, apply powder or cornstarch to

them to absorb any moisture of the day.

TIP # 9:

Regardless of how embarrassing it may be to you to clean his genitals, they must be washed and rinsed thoroughly to avoid rashes and possible sores from forming. If he doesn't qualify for a home health aide and you cannot bring yourself to do this, ask another family member.

It's up to you, but I never liked using latex gloves because I couldn't feel whether the soap was still on their bodies or not.

TIP # 10:

Use a very large, soft towel to cover him with as you are bathing him to preserve his dignity. Keep in mind how you would feel if you were naked for an extended period of time; helpless and at the mercy of a stranger, which is what you are or will eventually become as the dementia progresses.

TIP # 11:

Have him brush his teeth in the bathtub during the shower. This way, it makes less of a mess. We make it very easy for our residents by using battery operated toothbrushes.

TIP # 12:

To prevent a disastrous fall, dry all puddles of water immediately. Make sure you dry his hands before he reaches for the grab bars (dry them also) to steady

himself upon exiting the tub.

TIP # 13:

A large, terrycloth robe can be extremely beneficial for him to put on immediately after his bath. It helps to keep him warm while you tend to drying the rest of his body.

TIP # 14:

Stay on the lookout for agitation if you choose to use a blow dryer on his hair. The noise may upset or frighten him. If you do, make sure you hold it at least 12 inches from his scalp so you do not burn him. Remember, painful memories are among the last to go!

HOW TO BATHE A BED BOUND PERSON

A bed or sponge bath might be more appropriate in certain circumstances. If he has gotten to the point of being bed bound, more than likely, he will have a home health aide who will come in 3-5 times a week and bathe him for you.

If he cannot sit up, is very heavy or semi-conscience, he will require a bed bath. If he gets hysterical in the tub or shower and grows increasingly combative, try a sponge bath but still taking care to leave him covered, exposing only the area you are bathing and keep him warm.

Make sure not to use regular soap as it is very hard to rinse thoroughly. Instead, use a no-rinse soap, available at most medical supply houses and pharmacies. Simply pour the directed amount into a small plastic basin filled with warm water. Use the washcloth to clean him and then dry one area at a time.

Change the bath water 3 times: (1) to clean his face and then upper body (2) to clean the back and genital area and (3) to clean his legs and feet.

BATH TIME CLOSE TO THE END OF LIFE

When you have been told that your LO is very close to passing away and/or is having a difficult time breathing or may be experiencing pain, you should not put him through any more discomfort than absolutely necessary. At this point, bathing is no longer necessary; neither is turning him around the clock.

You might want to use a warm cloth to wipe his face and head, but a full bed bath would only be more traumatic than beneficial to him.

When he is in what is called "the active dying process", he will stop voiding urine and feces because he has already stopped taking in fluids and food. Diaper changes will cease. If he does urinate or have a slight bowel movement, be very gentle as you change him. If you notice that any remaining urine is turning dark red, do not be alarmed. It is a normal part of the dying process.

It is not an easy feat; getting over to the other side. Make his last few hours or days on this earth as comfortable as you possibly can.

HAIR CARE

When your LO is in the early stages of dementia, it is easier to take him to the hairdresser than to attempt doing it yourself at home.

Most elderly women have always taken pride in having their hair freshly rolled and styled weekly and these memories are among the last to go. Men, as well, have gone to the barbershop for their haircuts most of their lives.

If your LO is a woman and is not lying in bed most of the time, it is important that you continue this weekly ritual as long as possible.

When the dementia progresses and she is in bed, it is our recommendation that you see to it that she receives a very short haircut, stylishly done, to prevent matting on the back of her head. It is also easier to keep clean when it is short. At this point, vanity takes a back seat to practicality. By the same token, men need the same care.

Both men and women need their eyebrows to be trimmed back. Women need facial hair removed as soon as it is visible. For ears, eyebrows, nape of the neck hair and light facial hair, purchase the battery operated hair trimmers like Micro-Touch in your local pharmacy. They are quick, silent and great for the hard to get to places.

We have always had a hairdresser come to our home for a beauty day a few times a month. You can too. Just call one of your local beauty shops or haircut salons and ask one of the girls if they would like to make a few dollars on their day off by coming over and servicing your LO. Find a shop close to your home and maybe she could stop by on her way home from work.

We pay $10.00 for a cut and $30.00 for a perm. The hairdresser gets to keep all the money and will usually jump at the opportunity.

How do you shampoo a bed-bound patient? Purchase a no-rinse shampoo! All you have to do is pour it on his head (I usually warm it up in the microwave for a few seconds, but make sure that it is not too hot) and rub it in, then towel dry and style. It is that simple.

With the right supplies and equipment that are on the market in this high-tech day and age we live in today, it is not difficult to keep your LO well-groomed and clean with a little creativity and care.

SHAVING

Shaving your LO can be especially awkward if you are doing it yourself. If you have a home health aide, she will probably shave him three times a week. In between the days she comes, you can elect to either shave him yourself or let it go. If he gets agitated when shaved, it really wouldn't hurt to allow his beard to grow out and then keep it trimmed.

Men have new growth daily and need to be shaved more often than they care to if they have dementia. Some of the reasons your male LO objects to being shaved (if he does) and tips to help both of you are as follows:

PLAN OF ACTION!

TIP # 1:

The water is too cold or too hot. Prepare the temperature of the water as if you were giving a baby a bath.

TIP # 2:

There are too many distractions in the room. Do not have the television or stereo on while you shave him. Shave him in a quiet, small, well-lit room. If possible, do not have anyone else in the room. Other people moving around or talking could create confusion.

TIP # 3:

The razor is not sharp enough and it pulls on the facial hair causing pain and razor burn. Make sure you use a new disposable triple blade razor each time you shave him. Use a gel-based shaving cream that produces a good lather.

TIP # 4:

Never use soap as this tends to dry the skin.

TIP # 5

The upward strokes or haphazard strokes are uncomfortable for him. Instead, try downward strokes.

TIP # 6:

The aftershave lotion you use stings his face. Use a non-alcohol aftershave lotion for sensitive skin so it will not sting his face. The reason men use the lotion is that it helps to close the pores and soothe the skin.

TIP # 7:

He just doesn't like the whole process of a wet shave. In this case, invest in the best electric shaver on the market. Consumer Products can give you the current ratings and statistics but try and get the quietest shaver so the noise doesn't upset or frighten him. An electric shave is faster and less messy. Still, use the after shave lotion on him when you are through and clean the appliance after you use it every time so the blades remain sharp.

TIP # 8:

If shaving is still too traumatic for your LO, let

his beard grow out. It will be easier for both of you if you simply keep it trimmed. Many times I have trimmed the beards of our residents in their sleep to avoid all movement and confusion. It may be uncomfortable for some of your family members to get used to seeing him "hairy" but all that really matters is that he is clean and comfortable.

I have tried using depilatory cream but still haven't found one that removes the stiff facial hair completely and found it to irritate the skin anyway.

For hair in the ears, nose and back of the neck, you can pick up a nasal MicroTouch at almost any pharmacy. It is a handy little tool that emits very little noise and is also perfect for women's facial hair.

Trial & error will win out when it comes to shaving. Do not give up. Rah-rah, shish-boom-bah, fellow caregiver!

ORAL CARE

Try and imagine if you no longer had the ability to brush your teeth or did not even think about it. Unless you had someone to remind you or do the brushing for you, what would your mouth smell like? Nasty thought, right?

Hopefully, you brush at least twice daily. Your LO requires the same care you do. Not only will his breath stay fresh but you will be eliminating harmful germs that could potentially lead to gum or tongue infection and/or mouth sores if left undone. Here are a few tips to approaching mouth care:

Plan of Action!

Tip # 1:

Ideally, the brushing is accomplished easiest in the shower. Whenever you shower him, do it there.

Tip # 2:

Let's say that your LO still needs limited assistance with brushing. Have his toothbrush ready with toothpaste already on it, paper cup and towel ready before you take him into the bathroom.

Tip # 3:

See if he can still brush effectively (in your opinion). If so, let him. If not, ask him to open his mouth so you can finish up.

Tip # 4:

If he is in the latter stages of dementia, cannot perform his own oral care and will not open up for you, simply place a paper cup to his lips. His reflex will be to open up to drink. Then quickly, but carefully, place the toothbrush or toothette inside and commence brushing. A toothette is a round paper stick with a small, flavored sponge attached. Be prepared for him to bite down on it and refuse to let go. If he does, gently pull his chin down until he releases it.

Tip # 5:

Do not expect him to rinse and expel if he is in the latter stages of dementia. Allow him to

.

swallow and consider yourself fortunate that you even got inside of his mouth at all

A NOTE ABOUT DENTURES:

Your LO's mouth still needs the same oral care if he wears dentures. Soak the plates at night or brush and set aside in a cup until the next morning. When brushing the plates, line the bottom of the sink with a washcloth to avoid breakage in case they slip and fall. Brush the gums and tongue just as you would the teeth.

If he stops wearing them, the gums will usually shrink and then, after a while, the dentures will not fit or stay in place as they once did. If this happens and you are both in agreement for him to cease from wearing them, do not panic. Leave the plates out and begin to prepare a soft diet. Examples:

1. mashed or baked potatoes

2. spinach

3. Jell-O. pudding

4. oatmeal

5. meat loaf

6. ice cream

7. grits

8. pancakes

9. eggs

10. pimiento cheese

11. Vienna sausages

12. tuna salad sandwiches

As your LO begins to decline, the wearing of dentures will

become much less important to you and to him. Our rule of thumb for bed bound, terminally ill patients, is to do whatever makes them the most comfortable. Do not insist on the dentures toward the end for vanity's sake alone.

NAIL CARE

Keep your LO's fingernails clipped way back and blunt. If he ever gets combative with you, you'll soon find out why! Be very careful not to nick the skin or cause him pain or that may be the one thing he never forgets and he will not allow you to clip them again.

If he is a diabetic, it would better to leave the clipping to his nurse's aide or doctor unless you have successful experience doing it yourself. Even a small nick that draws blood can get infected and lead to gangrene.

Remember that the utmost in precaution must be taken with a diabetic. If you do elect to groom his nails yourself, be sure you use an alcohol spray to sterilize the nail tools, your hands, (before you latex-glove them) and his hands before and after the procedure.

If you must use colored nail polish, use the one minute drying type to avoid a mess. Most of the time, we stick with a clear gloss because if it smudges, you cannot see it.

The best time to clean his nails is right after his bath so that it loosens and softens any dirt or food under his nails. This makes it easier to remove.

If feces or anything else gets under his nails and you aren't going to bathe him right away, soak his fingers in warm, soapy water before you attempt to clean them. Use a nail brush to loosen the matter and then proceed with a nail file to finish up. The bacteria and acid in feces can lead to infection and sore nail beds, so never leave the cleaning for later.

The feet are often a neglected part of hygienic care in the elderly. The same precautions should be observed when trimming the toenails as the fingernails.

Usually, the fingernails receive more attention, but all extremities demand great caution when coming in contact with sharp objects. If your LO has corns or calluses in addition to a diabetic condition, be sure to consult with his podiatrist before using over-the-counter products to remove them.

You need to look at his feet every day to make sure there are no sores or open blisters. If you find there are, call the doctor or his nurse immediately so they can advise you.

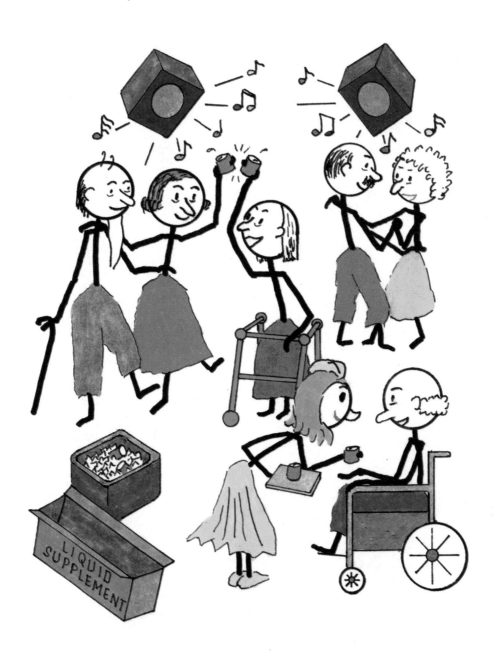

The House is Rockin

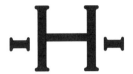

HOME SET-UP

THIS CHAPTER:

- **"The" Conversation**
- **Safety Precautions**
- **Bedroom**
- **Bathroom**
- **Kitchen**
- **Accommodations for Spouse**

HOME SET-UP

There can be many reasons for your moving your elderly parent in with you. See if you can identify with any of the following scenarios.

He isn't ready for a nursing home or assisted living facility but he cannot live alone anymore; it's just not safe. You found the stove left on several times you went over to check on him. He isn't taking his medication properly and sometimes, not at all.

The house is a mess. Dishes are stacked up in the sink and some of them have mold growing on them. Not only that, but when you ask him about a nasty looking burn on his hand, he tells you that he thinks it came from the hot water in the sink- he thought he was washing his hands in the cold water.

He is limping but he can't remember what happened but you suspect another fall. It's happening too frequently now.

He seems to have lost weight and when you look in his fridge and pantry, you are alarmed. The milk and orange juice are spoiled and the raw meat is rancid. That is all that you find in there. Nothing is in the freezer. The pantry is also bare and you wonder what he is eating.

You conclude that this dire situation calls for more than a sitter a few hours every day; he needs twenty-four hour supervision. Now, how do you tell him he is moving in with you?

"THE" CONVERSATION

Can you imagine being told you must move out of your home and that you have no choice in the matter? That you can only take a few of your things with you, but because of spacial limitations, the remainder will go into storage?

Before you allow your strong emotions to take over and go in to talk to him half-cocked, build your case for the move and commit it to writing in proposal form. Your priority should be to major on the advantageous elements; not the problem with him remaining in his home. For example:

Don't say:
"You left the stove on three times. I can't trust that you'll do it again and burn the house down with you in it!"
Instead, say: "Just think Dad, I'll be making your favorite meals like mom used to make for you. I'm going to make you feel so pampered!"

Don't say: "You can't even remember to wash the dishes, Dad. You're living like a pig and I can't put up with it anymore."
Instead, say: "Not only will you be eating well, Dad, but you won't have to clean up the kitchen. If you want to cook, I'll be your assistant!"

Don't say: "I can't trust you to live alone anymore. You have been depressed. You think I don't see it but I notice everything that is different about you."

Instead, say: "You know how often you ask me to come over because you have missed me so much? Well, we are going to be able to be together all the time now! We will have time to go through the photo albums, play checkers like we did when I was young and you can spend more time with your grandchildren. It's a dream come true for all of us!"

Don't say: "How can you expect not to waste away? Look at all the weight you have lost recently. You haven't gone grocery shopping in a long time and you don't have anything to eat in your house."

Instead, say: "With our living together Dad, you can help me do the grocery shopping and we can get your favorite foods, come back and fix them. How does that sound?"

Don't say: "You don't even think about me! I have a life too. I don't have time to keep on coming over here day after day but if I don't, I sit at home and worry about you. You aren't being fair."

Instead, say: "You won't have to wait for me to come over anymore. Whatever you need, we'll be able to do it for you much faster now."

Now that you understand how to keep the conversation positive, let us share a few tips on getting from point A to point B and get him moved in immediately:

PLAN OF ACTION!

TIP # 1:

Suggest that you both try it out for a few weeks or a couple of months. Keep it open-ended. If you make it sound permanent, he will feel that all power to choose his destiny will be taken away from him. It will take time to get used to living with each other, so be patient and tell him to do the same.

TIP # 2:

Plan a specific date for the move with his agreement. Whether it's in two days or two weeks, get out a calendar and write it down. Then put the calendar on the wall so he can look at it every day. If you do this, he will be able to accept it better emotionally.

TIP # 3:

Enlist the positive support and re-enforcement from other family members. Have them call him and talk about the benefits of moving in with you.

TIP # 4:

Plan a clean-up day with any members of the family willing to roll up their sleeves. Barbeque something outside while you work. Have your parent keep busy by providing him with some zip-lock bags and plastic shoe boxes and begin sorting out things in their drawers. If he's able, have him make a list of things to take with him to your house. He will feel more natural about it all when people he loves are surrounding him and making it a family effort.

TIP # 5:

If possible, let him choose the color of paint for his new room and then let him help paint it. Take him shopping for a new comforter to match the color of the room. Help him decide where his things should go.

TIP # 6:

Write down a list of house rules before he comes that everyone follows in the house. Post them in each room so he doesn't feel singled out. Go over them with him the first or second day he is there.

TIP # 7:

This is going to be quite a role reversal for both of you. Probably the last time you lived together, he was the head of the household and you had to obey his rules or suffer the consequences. He needs to understand, if he's able to, that although you are going to have a lot of fun, you need compliance with the established order already in place in your home. Talk to him about this when you go over the house rules.

Be sensitive to the possibility that he might be embarrassed about his dependence on you now, whereas you used to look up to him for advice and leadership.

If he has dementia, you probably won't have as much of a problem in this area because he will be dependent on you and will be relieved, subconsciously, to have decisions being made for him.

TIP # 8:

He will need a calendar in his room to keep track of his outside activities. If he makes his own doctor appointments, you will need to know about them, so tell him to be sure and write them on your home calendar as well. If you are making the appointments, you write them on both calendars.

TIP # 9:

Everyone needs their own space and privacy respected- everyone. Teenage boys are extremely territorial as they are going through puberty and need to be considered. When they have their friends over, there is an area in the house they feel comfortable letting their hair down in to play video games etc. Girls aren't as territorial but need their privacy and to know that you care about their feelings. If this is your parent, enlist the full support of your spouse and value his/her opinion regarding all decisions. Don't leave him out. You will all need to make adjustments but who says it can't be done with compassion, empathy and love.

TIP #10:

Before your parent comes to live with you, hold a family meeting- make sure everyone in the house is in attendance except your parent. Talk about the following topics, allowing everyone to speak their mind and give their suggestions and opinions:

- Privacy concerns
- Bathroom schedules
- Sharing space
- Pitching in to spend time with him
- The noise level adjustment
- House rules
- Individual duties/tasks
- Nail down a date for the next family meeting which will include your parent next time.

TIP # 11:

There are a number of details which must be attended to with your parents' house when they will no longer be living there. Make a checklist similar to this one.

1. Newspaper delivery
2. Utilities
3. Security measures- locks secured etc.
4. Mail forwarding
5. Keeping up lawn care
6. Neighbors alerted to keep an eye out
7. Perishable food taken with him

Okay. Now, let's talk about setting up your home for the care of an emotionally, mentally or physically disabled adult.

SAFETY PRECAUTIONS

RUGS

The number one cause of falls in the elderly is throw rugs, so if you are going to care for your parent, get rid of them. They may be beautiful and go perfect with your décor but it isn't worth the risk of sending your loved one to the hospital.

SHOES

If your loved one is still able to walk at all, get them some light weight, non-skid shoes. They shouldn't be too bulky and should fit snugly so they don't flop around when they walk. In my opinion, Velcro has been the most important invention when it comes to shoe wear, for mothers and the elderly. We recently went to a local shoe store, SAS, and found the lightest weight, Velcro shoes with built-in arches that we've ever seen. Talk about comfortable and safe! By taking the time to find a good pair of shoes, you will help your loved have a more comfortable walking experience for a longer period of time.

House shoes, if not fit to the foot, can cause falls. If they like to walk around in sock-feet, make sure you buy them the ones that have the little strips of rubber attached to the soles. They are comfortable, machine washable and won't slip on the most slippery floors.

FLOOR SURFACES

Thick carpet and slick tile are accidents just waiting to happen. Install non-skid strips on the tile and replace the carpet if it causes him to stumble.

Smooth cement, when wet, is extremely slippery so take extra care if your loved one has occasion to be outside after a rain or when someone has watered the yard.

OTHER SAFETY HAZARD MEASURES

Make sure walkways are clear of clutter, plants, wires and unnecessary furniture. Survey your home for anything hanging in the path he may walk.

Install grab bars for him to use as he walks along halls and outside walkways.

If space permits, place a small high-backed bench in his room for him to put on his shoes and to help him dress. Make sure it's very sturdy.

Check all chairs in the house to make sure there are no loose screws or too wobbly.

Wheelchair brakes must be checked for tightness at least twice a year. Place a thick tape over any sharp edges of the wheelchair or the feet of the chair.

LIGHTING

The darker any area in your home, the more opportunity there is for him to fall. Bright lighting, recessed or aimed upward toward the ceiling is best. Avoid positioning lights that would tend to shine directly in his eyes or it might blind him and cause falls as well. Next to his bed, place a touch lamp to make it easier for him. Make use of nightlights in his room, bathroom, kitchen and anywhere else he might walk during the night so he can easily find the light switch. Replace the standard light switches with illuminated switches that are light sensitive. There are also sound activated lights you could install for optimum safety.

IF YOUR LOVED ONE FALLS

Why is it that the first thing someone does to try to help a person who has fallen on the floor, is to try to pick them up? Many times, this is the worst thing you can do. You can make a broken bone worse if you move them wrong. If it's a rib that is broken, you risk puncturing a lung.

If they have fallen in water, you may have to move them. In this case, use a dry towel to lay hold of an uninjured part of their body and enlist the help of another person to help move them.

Even if you have taken every precaution possible, your loved one may still fall. If this happens and it's a bad fall, in your opinion, call 911 immediately. You should have easy access to his personal information folder (Paperwork chapter) so you can answer their questions quickly.

Even if it's a minor fall, he could still have a broken bone that goes undetected. After he is secure and comfortable, call his doctor and report what happened and get his advice on what to do next. He may suggest that you take him in for x-rays or that you call his secretary for an appointment.

SETTING UP YOUR LOVED ONE'S BEDROOM

This room will be the most important room out of the entire house for your loved one. This will be his refuge; his resting place; his private place. Include him in the decorating plans to help him take possession of it emotionally. We are going to give you tips on bedroom set-up for the person who spends most or all of his time in his bed and another set of tips for the person who is more ambulatory (moves around more).

If your loved one can still walk around or manipulate his wheelchair, the bedroom is set up with them in mind; for their convenience. If he is bed-bound, it's set up for the caregiver's convenience.

PLAN OF ACTION!
BED-BOUND SET-UP:

TIP # 1:

If you have not enlisted the help of a hospice or home health agency, talk to your loved one's doctor to see if he qualifies. If so, they will provide the hospital bed. If not, ask the doctor to write the order for you to take to the medical equipment supply company he does business with so your loved one is more comfortable. If none of this works, you may need to purchase a used bed so check out the classifieds for a fully electric hospital bed. Don't get the one that moves by way of a crank or you'll soon have back trouble of your own!

TIP # 2:

Other medical equipment you may need is a bedside commode (if he doesn't use adult diapers), an over-the-bed tray, a gel mattress for the bed, a wheelchair and wheelchair pad. These are all great tools to make your job easier and your loved one more comfortable. Again, talk to your doctor or home health provider for these items if you need them.

TIP # 3:

You will need a medium size table to hold the following items:

- Baby wipes
- Moisture barrier ointment
- Stack of diapers
- Peri-wash
- Box of Kleenex
- Roll of paper towels
- Box of latex gloves
- Waterless shampoo
- Eucerin lotion-pump
- A plastic drinking cup and small pitcher of purified water
- A mouth cleansing tray for oral care

Order some hospital gowns from the medical equipment supply company to keep on hand. It can be very difficult to change someone with pants on in bed. The most important thing to consider with someone who is bed-bound is expediency, not vanity.

TIP # 4:

If your loved one stays in bed, you might want to consider having their hair cut short, especially in the back. This will help prevent it from matting and be easier to keep clean.

TIP # 5:

Rather than using regular

sheets, get some hospital bed sheets-they will fit better.

Tip # 6:

There will be more room for you to move around in if you put a small chest of drawers in his closet rather than out on the floor.

Tip # 7:

Keep an extra 4 pillows in the top of his closet. You'll need them later to help prevent pressure sores.

Tip # 8:

If room permits comfortably, place a small desk and a chair in a corner of the room. Nurses and aides will need this to write their notes on his chart.

Tip # 9:

Keep a couple of folding chairs handy for visitors.

Tip # 10:

Bring his favorite photos from home and make a family gallery on his walls.

Tip # 11:

Mount a television in a corner in his room for his easy viewing rather than wasting space on a counter type model.

Tip # 12:

He will need a waste paper basket with a lid for paper items. This should not be used for diapers. Soiled diapers should be bagged separately and taken outside to a trash receptacle.

Tip # 13:

Get a pole lamp with three lights on it. Keep the lamps aimed at the ceiling.

PLAN OF ACTION!
AMBULATORY ROOM SET-UP

TIP # 1:

Set up the size bed he is most comfortable in and as space permits. If his own bed from home fits, bring it for him to make him feel more at home.

TIP # 2:

Bring his favorite photos from home and make a family gallery on his walls. Let him choose which ones he wants to hang.

TIP # 3:

He will need a desk, chair and chest of drawers. If there is room, get him his own miniature fridge and keep it stocked with his favorite drinks.

TIP # 4:

A small waste paper basket is all he needs, but keep it out of the way so he doesn't trip over it.

TIP # 5:

He will need a bedside table with a touch lamp and a nightlight.

TIP # 6:

Keep his pants together and his shirts together in the closet so he can find what he wants easily.

THE BATHROOM PLAN OF ACTION!

TIP # 1:

Either install a handicap commode, which is higher than the standard toilet, or place grab bars around it so he can guide himself down to the seat easier.

TIP # 2:

If you can afford it, hire someone to take out the bathtub and have a handicap shower stall put in. Most have only a two inch lip on the floor to contain water. It's so much easier for your loved one to get in and out of.

Get one with a built-in, folding shower bench. The shower hardware has a convenient portable showerhead so the caregiver can easily rinse their loved one. There are also safety grab bars with a rough surface for him to hold on to.

Don't get a shower with a glass or plastic door. Use a vinyl shower curtain instead- it's safer.

TIP # 3:

Place a utility tower in the corner of the shower if it doesn't come with one built in. You can keep all items you will need to bathe your loved one on it.

THE KITCHEN
PLAN OF ACTION!

TIP # 1:

Clean out one area for your loved one's things like medications, pill crusher, pill cutter, special foods and dishes.

TIP # 2:

Keep some cooked frozen food on hand for company. You might need to whip up something to eat for an unexpected family group so be prepared.

TIP # 3:

If your loved one has dementia and you need to keep him out of the kitchen for safety reasons, install a child-proof gate at the door. You may have to place it midway in the door jamb so he can't get over it.

ACCOMMODATIONS FOR SPOUSE

Let's say both of your parents are living but the well parent is no longer able to care for the ill parent. They don't want to live apart and you are willing to care for both of them. Before you sign up for this monumental act of love and most difficult job, consider the following:

1. Do your parents get along well enough to live in the same room?
2. Does your well parent interfere with the care your ill

parent needs?

3. Are you going to have ample time to care adequately for both parents?

4. Do you have room for both parents?

5. Do both of your parents get along with your spouse and children or do you anticipate strife?

6. Have your children still living at home and your spouse agreed to have them both come and stay?

7. Have you investigated other living options and discussed it with them for their feelings about it?

If everyone is agreed to their coming to live with your family and they want to stay in the same room, set up two single beds or a single bed and a hospital bed.

Be sure to keep it all open-ended and whatever you do, don't sell their house yet; they may need it again in the future if things don't work out in your home.

Then again, everything may work out fine, so remain positive.

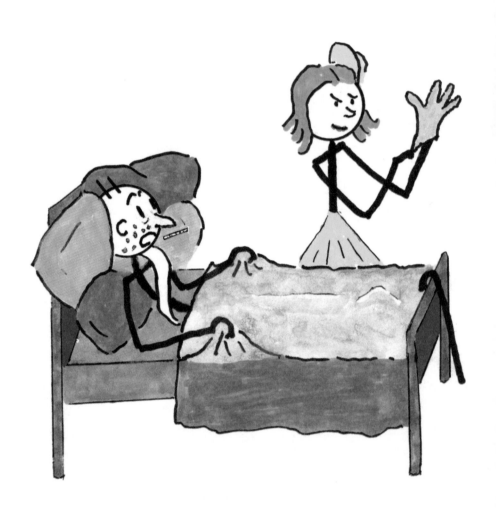

Love Will Keep Us Alive

I

ILLNESSES

THIS CHAPTER:

- **Constipation & Diarrhea**
- **Diabetes**
- **Fever**
- **Medication**
- **Pain**
- **Pneumonia & Other Breathing Problems**
- **Swelling**
- **Vomiting**

★ *Starr Calo-oy* ★

ILLNESSES

O ur elderly can be extremely susceptible to illness. If even the smallest signs of discomfort are ignored, it can be life threatening.

This chapter is not meant to cover these maladies in detail, but to enlighten the reader on their existence. Always consult your LO's doctor when you notice the first instance of the following ailments.

CONSTIPATION & DIARRHEA

Once upon a time, long ago, someone started an urban legend that if the elderly did not take boatloads of laxatives daily, they would become so clogged up that they would explode. They all seemed to buy it. That is why if your LO misses a bowel movement for one day, he panics and downs the laxatives.

Unfortunately, this causes constipation. When someone habitually takes laxatives to move their bowels, their body comes to rely on them, gets lazy and ceases to function naturally.

It is easier for a family caregiver to give in to their LO and give them their laxatives than to put up with their complaining but it is not healthy for them if they take them out of habit rather than true constipation.

When someone, regardless of his age, is constipated, it can be very painful. Hemorrhoids can develop quickly and the burning and itching that comes along with the pain can create fear. Anyone who has experienced this can relate and be sympathetic.

Constipation may be caused by a wide variety of conditions. Certain medications, hormonal problems, a lack of water and dietary habits can be the underlying culprits.

PLAN OF ACTION!

TIP # 1:

You need to check the side effects on the information sheet that comes with your LO's medications from the pharmacy. If constipation is one of them, ask his doctor for an alternative.

TIP # 2:

Invest in a book on a high fiber diet and begin to slowly change your LO's eating habits. Make sure he drinks 8 glasses of water daily and do not allow him to eat foods, like cheese, that are known to cause constipation.

TIP # 3:

Diarrhea can be just as uncomfortable. If your LO has it for longer than a week or it seems to be chronic, he could become dehydrated. If this happens, talk to his doctor. He will probably prescribe some medication to stop the loose bowels but stay on top of it.

If he doesn't seem to be getting any better after one day, call the doctor back and see if he can be seen immediately. The doctor might want to run some tests on him because diarrhea can be a symptom of a major health problem such as colon cancer, impaction or diabetes.

If he is lactose intolerant and gets a hold of a dairy product such as milk, cheese or cream, he could become very ill and diarrhea could start within an hour of ingestion.

If your LO wears adult briefs and has diarrhea, make sure you change him as soon as he has a bowel movement or he will get chapped from the acid and impurities in the feces. Also, use A&D Ointment on his anus to prevent soreness.

DIABETES

When our bodies do not create enough insulin or it fails in it is process of producing its insulin and sugar builds up in our blood, diabetes is the result.

Type 1 diabetes requires insulin injections and is usually apparent from birth. Type 2 diabetes, which makes up 90% of all diabetic cases, can usually be controlled with a proper diabetic diet and pills, in the early stages, but not always.

Those who are obese and do not exercise regularly are at high risk. When your LO has his annual checkup, his doctor will probably check his blood sugar.

Some of the symptoms of a diabetic are:

- Excessive thirst
- Persistent hunger
- Frequent urination
- Irritability
- Fatigue
- Clamminess

If you feel your LO is exhibiting the symptoms of diabetes, call his doctor and make an appointment.

FEVER

A fever usually means there is an infection of some kind in the body. There are so many illnesses in which a fever is present that it would be dangerous to your LO for you to guess and try to treat it yourself. Therefore, if your LO has a temperature, call his doctor immediately and he will ask you what the symptoms are and then advise you.

MEDICATION

Even if your LO does not have dementia, he still needs help taking his medication if you are having to take care of him.

PLAN OF ACTION!

TIP # 1:

If he is taking many meds each day and a new one has just been prescribed, ask his doctor or the pharmacist to review the compatibility of all medications involved. Many times, there are side effects when the chemical components in different drugs collide such as dizziness, constipation, confusion, agitation, tremors, insomnia and drowsiness. If you notice any unusual behavior in your LO, call his doctor immediately.

TIP # 2:

You can purchase a small plastic container with built-in compartments for each day of the week, four times a day, to fill with your LO's medications so you can keep track of them easier. Taking this measure can prevent a disastrous episode of double dosing which could prove to be fatal. We get the "Medi-Set" brand available at most pharmacies. If you fill them weekly, it will take the memory element out of it-

even for you!

TIP # 3:

Do not leave his pill bottles lying around. After you have filled his medication container, place the bottles in a zip-lock bag and put it away so no one can get to it.

TIP # 4:

Overmedicating is a major problem with the elderly, especially for those who have dementia. It can take many attempts at trying different behavior-modifying medications and dosages before a doctor finds one that works. As your LO's primary caregiver, it will be your responsibility to watch out for side effects and to use common sense when administering his medications.

TIP # 5:

It is equally important that you stay on top of getting your LO in to see his physician for regular check-ups. He may require a different dosage and/or medication or combination to treat his current condition.

TIP # 6:

If your LO has had no problem in the past with incontinence, begins a new medication or different dosage of a same medication and begins to have "accidents", tell his doctor about it. It could be the medicine. The elderly have the same delicate balance as a baby and it can be upset by even the smallest change. Do not let too much time go by before you call him. If you wait too long, the incontinence could become irreversible and introduce a new problem that could have otherwise been prevented.

TIP # 7:

Even over-the-counter medications can present a problem. Always ask the pharmacist before introducing something new to his system. When you talk to him, be sure to go prepared. Provide him with a list of your LO's current medications so he can make an assessment.

When the instructions on the bottle say to take the pills with food, comply. If you do not, it could cause your LO to vomit or worse.

TIP # 8:

Certain meds are to be taken in the a.m. and others in the evening. Always follow instructions to the letter.

TIP # 9:

Invest in a pill crusher and a pill splitter. If your LO feels uncomfortable taking a whole pill, try crushing it and putting the powder in his food. Do what works for you.

PAIN

When your LO complains of pain, ask him the following questions:

- Where is the pain located?
- Does the pain throb consistently or does it feel like sharp, knife-like jabs?
- On a scale of 1-10, 1 being the least and 10 being the most severe, where is your pain?

When you call his doctor or nurse, be ready to answer their questions. They will most likely ask if he has fever, when the last bowel movement was, what medications is he on currently, if he is crying, dizzy or vomiting. Then tell them the specifics regarding the pain itself based on your LO's answers when you asked him the above questions.

If your LO is ambulatory, the doctor will want to see him in his office so set up an immediate appointment.

If your LO has home health, the nurse should be notified and she will come right away. After an evaluation, she will consult with the doctor, usually right from your home by phone and he will order the appropriate medication for him.

One of the most common concerns that we have seen family members have regarding pain medication, is their LO will become addicted to it. If their LO is terminally ill, what does it matter? All that matters is they are comfortable and not suffering.

Another worry is that their LO is sleeping too much. If the only way your dying LO can be free from pain is to sleep right now, how can you deny him the dosage which will take the torment away?

If your LO does not have dementia and is experiencing considerable pain, you should still ask yourself the above questions.

We aren't saying that overmedicating is not a problem but what good does it do them to be fully awake and in excruciating pain?

There can be many reasons for a person to have pain and it takes a professional to make that determination.

Do not allow your opinions to stand in the way of your LO's relief. Get them the help they are depending on you to provide as their caregiver.

PNEUMONIA & OTHER BREATHING PROBLEMS

When people of any age and with any medical problem become bed-bound, they are prime candidates for breathing disorders. The angle at which they are lying combined with the lack of movement can cause can cause a lung infection because of bacteria. Everyday, ordinary motion keeps all of us healthy, so when we become sedentary, it can reverse our state of health very quickly.

It is bad enough not to be able to breathe but when a

dementia patient develops complications in this area, they become totally disoriented, more confused, may stop eating and drinking altogether and can become practically comatose. Their system is so very delicate and fragile that any slight imbalance can throw them off completely.

Also, contrary to popular belief, people do not die of Alzheimer Disease or any other type of dementia. They die from medical complications which arise from dementia. Pneumonia is one of them.

In the latter stages of dementia, people become bed-bound and unless their caregiver sees to it that they are turned from side to side, mucous, and other liquids, can settle in their lungs and cause an infection.

Dementia affects the brain, which in turn can affect our swallowing mechanism. When this happens, anything that is swallowed may not always go into their stomach. It may go into his lungs instead. Once a foreign object enters the lungs, the body tries to rid itself of it by coughing it up. If they are too weak to cough, it can result in volumes of phlegm going into the lungs.

If a liquid continues going into the lungs, it can cause your LO to develop pneumonia.

Pneumonia is characterized by fever, coughing and difficulty breathing. It can be treated by the aggressive use of antibiotics, diuretics to help dry up the fluid out of the lungs and the pushing of fluids so as to prevent dehydration. If his saturation level is too low, the doctor may order oxygen therapy.

If your LO develops swallowing problems and chokes on liquids, try using a liquid thickener such as "Thickett". This non-flavored powder can be used in any beverage to make it easier to swallow.

When a person gets pneumonia, it can cause them to become very confused and/or non-verbal.

If you suspect your LO has pneumonia, try to keep his head elevated, give him a very small amount of water at a time unless he chokes, and if he does, cease the fluids. Call the doctor or his nurse immediately.

SWELLING

As we age, we slow down. Our circulatory system and metabolism slows as well. If you notice your LO has swollen ankles or feet, it could indicate water retention.

Congestive heart failure is common among the elderly population and one of the first signs is swelling. Get him to the doctor immediately if the swelling is consistent. This can be very painful for him. Until the time of his appointment, his doctor will probably tell you to keep his feet elevated and use ice packs and ibuprofen for the pain.

VOMITING

Needless to say, if your LO begins to vomit, call the doctor, the home health agency or his nurse.

Keep his head and shoulders elevated or turn him to one side to prevent asphyxiation.

Do not give him anything by mouth, and that includes fluids because they may come right back up unless his doctor advises you to do so.

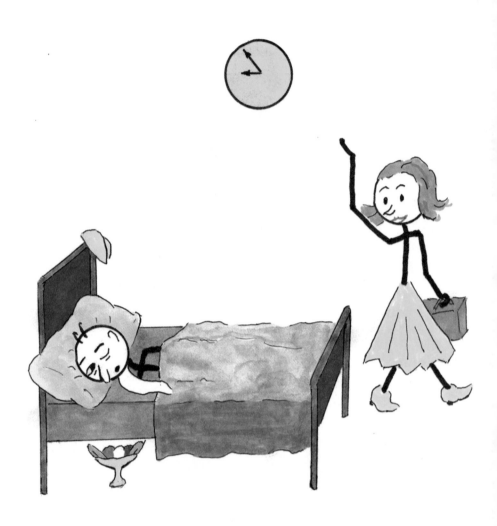

9 to 5

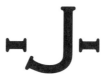

JOB/CAREER

THIS CHAPTER:

- **Family and Medical Leave Act**
- **Stages the Family Goes Through**
- **An Alternative to Consider**

JOB/CAREER

Working outside the home at a full time job while caring for an aging, disabled parent can be one of the most challenging situations a person can go through.

Your already jam-packed schedule is suddenly toppled the moment you realize that you have a life and death situation that must be addressed with your LO.

Time doesn't stand still. There are still

children to care for, a spouse who needs you and an employer whose patience is sure to run short if there are too many more absences. What do you do? Hopefully, in this chapter, we can give you some advice that will change your life for the better and help you get back to sanity.

FAMILY AND MEDICAL LEAVE ACT

Why don't we start out with some good news for you? The following information was taken directly from the Department of Labor website. I am providing it for those boomers out there who are not computer savvy! If you are and want to look it up on your computer, go to www.dol.gov/elaws

Did you know that if you have worked for an employer for 12 months or longer (actual working hours totaling 1250) and the employer has 50 or more employees and you meet the following criteria, that you are entitled to request a FMLA leave of absence.

HOW MUCH TIME OFF MAY
I HAVE UNDER THIS ACT?

"If you are an "eligible" employee, you are entitled to 12 weeks of leave for certain family and medical reasons during a 12-month period."

THIS LEAVE CAN BE USED TO CARE FOR:

"An employee's spouse, children (son or daughter), and parents are immediate family members for purposes of FMLA. The term "parent" does not include a parent "in-law". The terms son or daughter do not include individuals age 18 or over unless they are "incapable of self-care" because of mental or physical disability that limits one or more of the "major life activities" as those terms are defined in regulations issued by the Equal Employment Opportunity Commission (EEOC) under the Americans with Disabilities Act (ADA)."

PAID OR UNPAID LEAVE?

"The FMLA only requires unpaid leave. However, the law permits an employee to elect, or the employer to require the employee, to use accrued paid leave, such as vacation or sick leave, for some or all of the FMLA leave period. When paid leave is substituted for unpaid FMLA leave, it may be counted against the 12-week FMLA leave entitlement if the employee is properly notified of the designation when the leave begins."

ELIGIBILITY

"Employees are eligible to take FMLA leave if they have worked for their employer for at least 12 months, and have worked for at least 1,250 hours over the previous 12 months, and work at a location where at least 50 employees are employed by the employer within 75 miles.

The 12 months do not have to be continuous or consecutive; all time worked for the employer is counted. The 1,250 hours include only those hours actually worked for the employer. Paid leave and unpaid leave, including FMLA leave, are not included."

CAN I LOSE MY JOB BY TAKING ADVANTAGE OF THIS ACT?

"It is unlawful for any employer to interfere with, restrain, or deny the exercise of any right provided under this law. Employers cannot use the taking of FMLA leave as a negative factor in employment actions, such as hiring, promotions or disciplinary actions; nor can FMLA leave be counted under "no fault" attendance policies. Under limited circumstances, an employer may deny reinstatement to work - but not the use of FMLA leave - to certain highly-paid, salaried ("key") employees."

There is much more information available on the website or if you want to write to the Department of Labor at:

U.S. Department of Labor
Frances Perkins Building
200 Constitution Avenue, NW
Washington, DC 20210

STAGES THE FAMILY
GOES THROUGH

There are so many variables to address in regard to holding down a job and the responsibilities of an aging parent, so I have chosen one of the most common.

The following is a fictitious story to illustrate the 8 stages Ruth goes through before she realizes she needs help. Denial coupled with guilt on the part of a well-meaning family, can add up to an early death for a LO.

In this story, Ruth does not have the support of any other family members or much money to hire outside help and either does her mother. She really has no other choice but to place her mother in an alternate living facility.

Unfortunately for her mother, she delays the inevitable decision almost too late.

I have already provided a solution for the working family caregiver who enlists the family's support. In our chapter on "Family" in "The Family Gathering" section, she keeps her job and her LO in her home. Please refer to that chapter for details and tips.

Let me set the following scene for you. I will use the words "mother" for the elderly LO and "Ruth" for the daughter.

Mother stays at her own home by herself and refuses to let anyone come in to help her. She can no longer stay in her own home alone, due to safety reasons, but Ruth cannot bring herself to step in and force the move. (Again, this story refers to

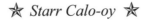
male or female LO's).

☐ STAGE 1 or "CALLER ID ANYONE?"

Mother begins calling Ruth at work much more often for unimportant things. Ruth loves her mother and doesn't ask her to stop calling; she even feels guilty at the mere thought of turning away her mother who has always been there for her all these years.

☐ STAGE 2 or "SECRETARY OF THE YEAR!"

As time goes by, Ruth notices that mother is missing her doctor appointments. She has her utilities cut off one by one as she forgets to pay them. Ruth takes over mother's finances and opens an account at the bank in both their names. She really doesn't think anything of it, even though, unknowingly, she has just added more stress to her already jam-packed lifestyle.

Ruth sets up a database on her computer and buys a program so she can keep track of mother's bills. She does this, in addition to her own family's bills, so now she is doing double the work. She also begins to keep track of her mother's various doctor appointments, such as her psychiatrist, neurologist, general physician, and her eye doctor.

Ruth not only has to make these appointments, but also has to call to remind mother to go one day in advance and then also on the day of the appointment, because mother will forget otherwise.

After the appointment, Ruth has to call and talk to the nurse to see what the doctor said because mother doesn't remember. Ruth has to make sure mother has picked up the prescriptions at the pharmacy so she makes a follow up call to them as well, after each doctor visit.

She then has to fill her mother's medi-set for the week and check daily to make sure mother is taking her medication. This all takes a great deal of time and effort not to mention patience, which Ruth is already starting to run short of.

☐ STAGE 3 or "THE UNPAID AND UNAPPRECIATED CHAUFFER"

Mother starts denting and scratching her car and sometimes gets lost going places and can't find her way back home. Sometimes while her mother is out shopping, she forgets where she parked and Ruth has to handle the situation with store security.

Ruth wrestles with the monumental decision to take mothers keys away from her, but finally gives in when mother forgets to put the garage door up before parking the car in it. Mother is furious with Ruth because she thinks Ruth is treating her like a child and she wants to drive, so their relationship is strained.

Ruth is determined to make sure her mother is safe and that matters now more than anything else does. However, Ruth has added to her already intense workload, taking mother to the grocery store, and it seems that mother needs to go daily because she is always forgetting something.

She must take her to the pharmacy, restaurants, beauty

salons, doctor appointments and take her clothes to the cleaners. By this time, Ruth is now going to mother's house at least once daily.

She does all of this on her time off from her full-time job and between this and caring for her own husband and family, burnout begins to become apparent. She is tired most of the time and feels pulled in every direction - trapped.

The phone calls at work escalate and now mother is also calling her in the middle of the night as well. Ruth often feels like ripping that phone out of the wall. Mother has lost touch with night and day, but Ruth can't bring herself to turn off the ringer at night. After all, that would make her feel even guiltier than she already does.

☐ STAGE 4 or "THE MAID"

Mother's lack of good hygiene is beginning to show. Ruth has to bathe mother every other day but they fight each time because mother refuses to get into the shower. Ruth also has to keep up her nails and hair.

She is astonished at how dirty the house is now because mother always kept an immaculate home. Mother rarely cleans it now-she even throws trash on the floor. The house even smells of urine. There are dirty dishes in the sink and laundry is stacked up everywhere. Ruth has to put the trash out on trash days now. She is also surprised at how dangerous a home can be.

☐ STAGE 5 or "THE EMPLOYMENT COUNSELOR"

Her mother is beginning to fall regularly so Ruth tries to get someone to stay with mother a few hours a day. When she finally convinces mother to allow it, she finds that it's very expensive and there are still many unsupervised hours, so it really isn't worth it.

She puts an ad in the local newspaper, and then spends countless hours screening people on the phone, checking references, background checks, bonding agencies and past employers.

Over the course of several weeks, she finally makes appointments with 3 people to interview in person. One person doesn't show up, another has health problems of her own that she failed to disclose over the phone and the last one raised the fee from what she originally told Ruth she would accept.

Ruth feels she has no more time to invest in her search, so she agrees to hire the last one interviewed. When the sitter takes her day off, she doesn't return, isn't answering her phone and evidently has quit, without notice. Memories of all the hours that were put into finding a supposedly reliable and dependable sitter flood Ruth's mind and she feels the sting of hopelessness.

Depression begins to set in. Ruth feels she has nowhere else to turn for advice, so she asks mother's doctor who suggests a nursing home. She is suddenly overwhelmed by the guilt phantom at the mere thought of taking mother out of the home she grew up in, so instead, she puts off the decision and

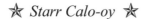

continues to do all of the work herself.

☐ STAGE 6- "FLORENCE NIGHTINGALE TO THE RESCUE"

Just when Ruth thinks it couldn't possibly get worse, disaster strikes. Mother has a bad fall this time and it is estimated that thirteen hours went by before she was discovered.

She is hospitalized with a broken hip and requires surgery. Ruth talks to her employer and he agrees to let her take her vacation time. Ruth and her family had planned to go to Hawaii for two weeks this summer but that's out now. All she can think of while her mother is on that operating table is she should have made the decision to take her out of her home sooner.

When mother is out of surgery and in recovery, Ruth goes home to pack a bag. She has permission to stay in her mother's room at the hospital. As the anesthesia wears off, you can hear the wails and cries all down the hall emanating from her mother's room. Ruth waits on mother hand and foot regardless of how outrageous the demands.

She gets very little sleep and her own family at home is beginning to fall apart. Ruth can't help the kids with their homework (and their grades are beginning to show it), be there to cook, do her laundry, clean her house and the relationship between herself and her husband is starting to become strained.

Her mother is released from the hospital after a ten-day stay and sent to a nursing home for rehabilitation. The doctor tells her that she will be in rehab for about a week but that Ruth needs to make plans to either leave her there permanently or find another place to take care of her because she cannot stay alone any longer.

□ STAGE 7 or "GUESS WHO'S COMING TO DINNER?"

Ruth, now surrounded by the guilt phantom, believes she can fight it off by moving mother in with her. Mary thought that the home health agency could help while she was at work but found that the nurse's aide only comes three times a week for forty-five minutes each visit but for only three weeks.

Ruth has already used up her vacation time so she uses her one-week of sick leave to seek other options. Sheer necessity temporarily overrides the guilt where the stigma of nursing homes is concerned, so she settles on one. When her mother does not make the adjustment, her doctor makes another suggestion; a personal, residential care home.

He tells her if she can find a good one, it will have a full-time, live-in staff to provide twenty-four hour care for her mother and that the average staff-to-patient ratio is about two to one. She will live in a home atmosphere with home cooking and most importantly, it will provide a break from all of the guilt she has taken on herself. She can get back to living her life again with her own family and know in her heart that she has done the best for her mother.

□ **STAGE 8 or "MASSACRE OF THE GUILT PHANTOM"**

Ruth calls from the list that her doctor has provided of personal care homes in the area and makes several appointments. She interviews the owners in their homes and selects one, and then she moves her mother in a couple of hours and goes home to sleep *guilt free.*

There are many other components not mentioned here. The sequence of events may be different and it could easily have been a dad, wife, husband, sister or brother. She could have found a wonderful nursing home right off the bat but I tried to explore every obstacle possible for your consideration.

The point I want to make is that guilt builds upon guilt and Ruth should have given herself credit for trying. Had she been able to see up the road what was coming, she could have skipped most of these stages. My greatest desire is that this story will help you to bypass most, if not all, of these painful stages on your journey to finding care for your loved one.

Remember, the guilt phantom will paralyze you and render your concentration ineffective. It brings on depression which triggers fatigue and you will need all of the energy you can muster to help your loved one while at the same time keeping up with your own responsibilities.

Over the years, we have seen many family members succumb to a heart attack or a stroke within two weeks of relinquishing the care of their loved one. It's almost as if their love for them and obligation to them served as a physical dam, keeping all severe health issues from manifesting. After they relaxed and the new caregiver had successfully alleviated the responsibility, their resistance to illness was seemingly gone.

Please don't put off this inevitable decision once you realize that it is time. You owe it to yourself, your own immediate family, your spouse and your loved one.

AN ALTERNATIVE TO CONSIDER

One of my favorite sayings is "Run toward the roar; not away from it." You might find the following suggestion exciting if you:

1. Have a heart for the elderly- in other words, if you like caring for them and they don't make you nervous or angry

2. If you aren't really attached to your present job, dislike the people you are working with or for and wish you were at home caring for your LO.

If you'd rather be at home, check with the local hospices and home health agencies to see if they could refer you to a family like yours who would rather have their LO cared for in a home-like environment. Many families cannot care for their

LO's any longer at home due to their own health problems but do not want them to go into a nursing home. If you are going to be home anyway, caring for your LO, why not care for one more, for pay?

At the print time of this book, the going rate for caring for someone with dementia at home is $3,500.00-$5,000.00. The care fee for someone well minded ranges from $$3,000.00-$4,000.00.

Each state has its own laws concerning the number of people you can care for without a license, but all states permit a minimum of 2 people and your own relatives do not figure into that number. In other words, for example, in the State of Texas, you can care for 3 people who are not related to you plus your own relatives without having a license. The purpose for a license is so you adhere to the fire departments rules for getting disabled people out of your home in case of fire. They figure that someone (in Texas for example) can get 3 people out of their home safely without having to purchase a sprinkler system or remodeling their house. Over 3, they would need to conform to the state rules for a personal care home license.

I am only talking about you being able to stay with your LO at home and still make the same, or close to the same, income you would make if you worked outside the home. There are many advantages to doing this.

1. You get to be with your LO.
2. You avoid the high cost of care.

3. You don't have to argue, fuss or fight with a boss who is not compassionate regarding time off to care for your LO or handle emergencies.
4. You control the quality of care your LO receives.
5. You can hire a live-in aide of your own to help you, for a fraction of what it would cost to place your LO in a care facility. This way you could train her to care for your LO the way you want and still be free to come and go with your family- you'd have a live-in sitter 24/7!

You are going to see more and more people retire from their jobs early to help their LO's in the future because eldercare is growing increasingly expensive. You may be asking yourself right now "But what about my benefits?" If you do the math and take in 2 residents, you can save a lot of money in the bank which will grow in interest and easily pay for your own benefits. Who said you need someone else to pay for them? Before you want to fight with me, as I said, do the math.

Anyway, it's not for everybody. I have always said you must be called of God to care for another human being. It cannot be solely because of money that you change your career to care for your LO- you must truly want to stay at home and care for him. Otherwise, you will grow impatient and angry eventually and feel as trapped as you felt in the job you left to care for him to begin with! Pray on it first- ask God what He thinks and then do it.

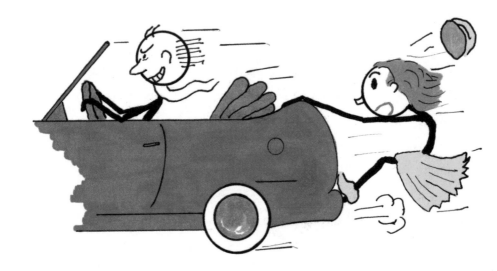

You Can Drive My Car

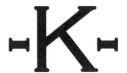

KEYS TO THE CAR:

HOW TO GET THEM BACK!

KEYS TO
THE CAR:

HOW TO GET
THEM BACK!

Your elderly LO is still driving and is beginning to exhibit signs of early dementia. You know that you have to intervene but you do not want them to get mad at you and you do not want to be responsible for an accident or worse. What do you do?

You are not alone in this dilemma. Every day that goes by, there are hundreds of adult children who have to make some very difficult and unpopular decisions for their elderly parents.

Some even have to fight their siblings on this issue making it more difficult. Hopefully we can help you with a few ideas. Just keep an open mind, even if you cannot see yourself doing what we suggest, and try them anyway. What do you have to lose? You might be pleasantly surprised!

In regard to driving, as a person gets older, his reflexes get slower, his peripheral vision decreases and his night vision dims. These obstacles are immensely compounded when the person starts getting confused as well.

A cognitively impaired person cannot respond quickly enough to a situation that demands a sudden and flexible response such as avoiding an accident. If they are on certain medications it can make matters even worse.

Also, as we age, our coordination is off, our balance and equilibrium begins to deteriorate. For a confused person, the fear of driving can cause them to have accidents instead of making them more cautious. They can become dizzy and even angry if they suffer from paranoia.

The reason that most elderly people fuss about relinquishing their driving is that they have enjoyed a great sense of independence all of their life when in control of their comings and goings. Men remember the pride they felt when they got their first car; the feel of their own set of keys in their pocket. This is a long term memory and usually one of the last to fade. For them to surrender their car and keys means a surrender of their manhood to them.

Then there is the universal problem we hear about on the news every day regarding an elderly person with dementia who has gone missing. They got into their car and got lost. Unfortunately, many of the homeless we see on the street are dementia patients who never found their way home.

Many times, they have made it all the way across the country and have forgotten their name and all other vital information that could identify them and help them get home if anyone took the time to care, which they do not. People just pass them by as if they are invisible mistaking them for derelicts.

This problem is much more prevalent than you may think. The saddest part of it all is that they probably have a worried family back home, a warm bed and lots of

TLC they are missing.

If you begin to suspect your LO is having difficulty driving, it is your responsibility to look into it further and put a stop to their driving. We realize this is a strong statement but consider the alternative. They could kill themselves and someone else if you do not. The question is how to accomplish this expediently without hurting their feelings.

Hopefully, you can use one of the following suggestions to keep everyone a little safer.

PLAN OF ACTION!

TIP #1:

Start going with him when he drives and keep an eye on the attention he pays to the following:

- The speed limit
- Stop signs

- If he misses cut-offs and exits
- The frequency and power with which he hits the brakes
- Staying in his own lane

You need to accompany him at least 5 times to get a good picture of how well he can drive. However, you may know after one trip. If, in your opinion, he should not be driving anymore, use one of the following tips.

TIP # 2:

Have his peripheral vision checked and consult with his eye doctor about his ability to drive safely. Speak with the doctor over the phone before the appointment to share your concerns with him. Ask him to help you by explaining to your LO that it is no longer safe for them to drive. When the news and advice comes from a doctor, it is received much more favorably than from a family member. If your LO will not listen to a physician, disable the car (discreetly) and/or take the car keys.

TIP # 3:

Make an appointment, if you haven't already, with a neurologist and have your LO thoroughly checked out. Enlist his help privately in advance.

TIP # 4:

If he has been driving a big car and the doctor, optometrist, and neurologist gives their approval for his continued driving, consider getting a smaller vehicle for him. It will be easier for him to park and help him to avoid clipping other cars. Make sure you get a car with power seats, locks, steering and brakes to make it as easy as possible for him.

TIP # 5:

This may sound strange, but introduce your LO to some simple video games! This can strengthen his motor responses and reflexes and help him to think faster. It is like exercising his brain. Do not laugh until you've tried it. If there are children in your family, enlist their help in teaching him.

Many games have 2 or more controllers and it could be a lot of fun and bonding for all involved.

You can accomplish more than improving his driving ability by doing this. He may not want to go anywhere if he really likes the games!

TIP # 6:

Make sure their seat belt fits and stress the

importance of never failing to wear it.

TIP # 7:

Have his car checked out. See to it that it is in good working condition.

TIP # 8:

Tell him that for the time being, he is never to drive at night (most elderly want to be home well before dark anyway), on the expressway or freeway, when it is raining or for long distances. You will have to resign yourself to check on him to make sure they are complying.

TIP # 9

Check out alternate transportation for him such as senior programs available in your area and others. (See the *"Transportation"* chapter of this book for tips)

TIP # 10:

As a last resort, if you cannot seem to be making any headway with stopping your LO from driving, report him to the Department of Motor Vehicles and tell them you would appreciate them allowing the report to remain anonymous. Just explain the situation and it wouldn't hurt if you got the doctor to write a letter of support stating that in his opinion, your LO should not be allowed to drive.

The rest of the family needs to be in one accord to support you when and if your LO runs to them and tells on you! After you have taken the above steps, you will have the "proof" needed to show the family that you tried many different ways to arrest the situation before taking other drastic measures.

On occasion, we have asked the doctor to speak with family members and reassure them they were making the right decision. Keep in mind that all of these suggestions are acts of love not of deprivation.

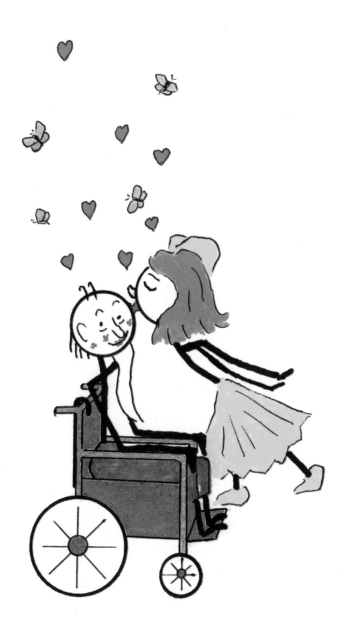

Kiss You All Over

-L-

LOVE, TOUCH
&
TENDERNESS

- "I'm loving her but she isn't feeling it!"
- "I haven't had any Love all Day!"
- How to Show Your Love

LOVE, TOUCH & TENDERNESS

What would the results be if a survey were taken from all of the people who know you? Would the majority say that you are a lovable, warm and caring person? Quite a point to ponder, is not it? When we are born, we are coddled, photographed, kissed, held and hugged. Everyone pays attention to us and the terms "adorable, cute and precious" all are used to describe us.

When we enter our pre-adolescent years, newer babies take the focus off of us.

As we age, our patience begins to diminish and we develop a lack of lenience for people and uncomfortable circumstances. We are tolerated by the youth who will someday take our place and then become less lovable.

In our prime (and on the journey up to it), we are on the go; moving at the speed of light and spending time with only those who can keep up with us. Even our children suffer from this practice. We sort of leave those slower than us behind in a trail of dust.

When you are attending your family reunions or family holiday parties, are your elders sitting it out on the sidelines? How many grand or great grandchildren take the time to really sit down and talk with them at length? How many people find them as interesting as the younger people?

The truth is that our elders have fascinating tales to tell and a wealth of experience for all of us to enrich our lives. We need to take the time to learn from them.

Everyone needs to be touched. Just imagine that you are 85 and all of your friends have passed away. The only family you have left is younger than you are. No one kisses or hugs you anymore, but you see others showing affection toward each other. The elderly experience this sadness every day because their family doesn't think about it.

We give love as a reward all our lives.

Sure, we greet each other with hugs sometimes, but unless someone has actually "done" something for us, they do not receive a deposit from our emotional bank.

When we believe that our elders are no longer able to contribute to us because they are old, the love they receive from us fades away.

Our goal with this chapter, is to make caregivers aware of the therapeutic healing properties in demonstrating love to their LO's.

We pray that you will use some or all of the tips in this chapter to begin expressing unconditional love and change not only your LO's life, but your own in the process.

"I'M LOVING HER BUT SHE ISN'T FEELING IT!"

I'm reminded of one summer day when our 2 smallest children, Khalea (daughter, 5) and Khaiyan (son, 7), had been playing outside. Khaiyan came into the house and made this statement to me, "Mother, I'm loving Khalea but she isn't feeling it!"

What a profound thing to say! He knew he wasn't making contact but desperately wanted to. Sometimes we feel the same emotions while caregiving for our LO's.

I changed hats, sat him down, and changed my speech and mannerisms to make contact with my remarkable son.

I said, "Son, people feel love in different ways. What love is to you doesn't always feel like love to others. You kind of have to be a love investigator and find out what actions show love to different people. For example, when Daddy brings home McDonalds to you and Khalea for supper without being asked, he is showing you love. He does something he knows means a lot to you sweetheart- that is love!"

Khaiyan finally grasped in his insightful, little mind that love meant different things to different people and still, to this day, looks into the hearts of those close to him to discover what love means to them.

"I HAVEN'T HAD ANY LOVE ALL DAY!"

Children are so expressive and raw. When Khalea's little emotional tank is running on empty, she will come and curl up in my lap and adamantly say "I haven't had any love all day!" What she's actually saying is "You haven't done a very good job of making me feel the love today Mother. Focus on me right now until I am satisfied that you love me."

She won't be denied. She is determined to get my attention and love right then and there. Children possess an innate need us to prove our love for them many times a day. After numerous, successful experiences of receiving acts and words of endearment toward them, they eventually need less proof on a daily basis. However, the need never goes away entirely, even if we live to be 100, we need the reassurance that those we love, love us too.

HOW TO SHOW YOUR LOVE

Touch is so underrated. This is one of our basic needs as human beings. God made us like this. From the time we are born into this world, most of us are coddled, held, touched, kissed and shown love in many ways.

Unfortunately, many elderly people experience touch deprivation. I truly believe many an elder has prematurely died because of the lack of touch in their lives brought about by a deep loneliness.

The extent of which the elderly receive touch is limited to the "hands-on", mechanical, daily caregiving chores. Affection usually doesn't play a part in average caregiving. Isn't this a shame? Many experts agree that as we get old, our need to be touched and nurtured lovingly increases. Instead, the practice of showing the elderly love decreases.

We endure many losses as we age, so in order to adequately compensate for the deficit, our souls emotionally and physically require demonstrative and tangible affection to remain healthy. We spend so much time on the physical care of our LO's, that we neglect their hearts.

If you are a "family" caregiver and this is your LO we are speaking of, there are many ways to speak the language of love. If you are caring for someone who is not blood related, we will show you how to teach their families through your example.

In either case, the most rewarding element of learning how to show love to someone is that you receive it back many times over.

PLAN OF ACTION!

TIP # 1:

If you LO is female, offer to brush her hair. You can show great affection in the way you brush it. When all the tangles are out, continue brushing and touching her head. Tell her how much she means to you as you do it.

TIP # 2:

A daily massage with soft music in the privacy of his room, with scented oil or lotion is a great way to express love through touch. If you take the time to do this, you will quickly see a dramatic peace come over your LO. This practice can help him to sleep better and heal faster than you can possibly imagine.

TIP # 3:

Even if your LO can feed himself, a loving thing to do for him is to occasionally pamper him by feeding him. Just be sure not to offend him by making him feel you are babying him.

TIP # 4:

If he is bed bound, ask the family to honor him at least once a week by eating dinner in his room so you can all eat together. He will feel very special if you do this. Fix his favorite food.

TIP # 5:

Interview him. Check out the chapter on "Life Stories" in this book and follow the instructions. Make him the star of his own life story! He will love reminiscing and you can play the finished DVD at family gatherings.

TIP # 6:

Hold monthly parties for him and invite the family to honor him.

TIP # 7:

Curl up in bed with him and watch a movie. Don't forget the popcorn.

TIP # 8:

If he is well enough, make a regular date with him to eat at his favorite restaurant each week.

TIP # 9:

If his spouse is not ill, surprise him by setting up a romantic dinner, complete with candlelight and sparkling wine.

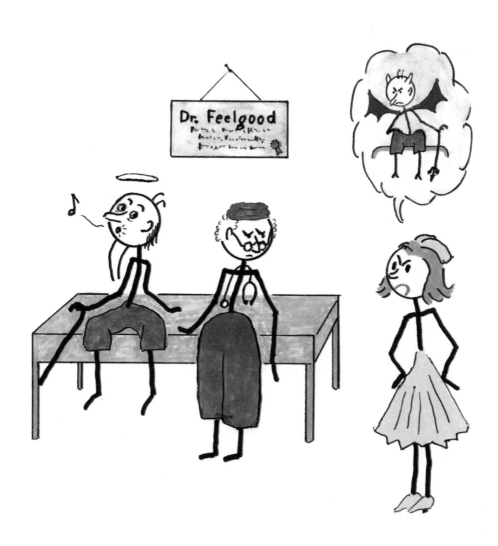

Make It with You

-M-

MEDICAL PERSONNEL

THIS CHAPTER:

- **Doctors**
- **Hospital stays**
- **Hospice nurses**
- **Home health aides**

MEDICAL PERSONNEL

Unless you have a background in medicine, it may seem to you that the medical workforce comes from a different planet! They have their own vocabulary, thought processes and circle of peers.

Many times, it can seem as if you are being ignored and it can be extremely frustrating since you are doing your best to honor your LO's wishes. Other family

**members are looking to you for
information. You need to get the attention
of the medical supervisors on your LO's
case so they can thoroughly explain the
situation to you. How do you accomplish
this?**

**We thought we'd include some tips in
this book, on dealing with this very special
group of people so you can feel more
comfortable while conversing with them.
This information can help you to make
wise decisions on his behalf and answer
your family's questions.**

DOCTORS

VISITS TO THE DOCTOR

We usually took our elderly LO's to the doctor for one of
two reasons; 1) for an annual check-up, or because
2) they were exhibiting symptoms of an illness.

Regardless of the reason (unless this is an emergency, and
then you need to dial 911), there are steps you can take which

will help you with the trip, start to finish and I'm going to share them with you in this chapter.

Let's start with the appointment. Before you call and make an appointment with the doctor's secretary, go through the following checklist and have these things handy while you talk to her:

1) Current medication list
2) The problem as you have observed it (if there is a problem)
3) State the necessity of not being made to wait.
4) Your LO's date of birth and insurance information.
5) Ask the doctors physical and e-mail addresses.
6) Your calendar

CURRENT MEDICATION LIST

It is a good idea for you to keep a manila file folder with all of your LO's important papers in it. On the outside of the folder, write his full name, date of birth, social security number, insurance information and doctor's name, number and after hours information. Among the important papers inside the folder, keep a sheet of paper with all of his current medication information listed for easy reference. The list should have the name of the medication, the dosage and the frequency he is to take it. Keep the list updated with any changes. This is very important.

DOCTORS REPORT

One of the most pleasant things you could do for your LO and his doctor is to send a report 2 days in advance describing the state of his health. The doctor has time to read and think about the best course of action and your LO will not feel slighted by your talking for him in the doc's presence.

Look at the following report example and then, design your own using this as a template. The names have been changed.

Report re: Mary Jones
Prepared by Starr Calo-oy
For Dr. Feelgood
4-6-06

Social Habits and Activities:

Mary has difficulty most of the time socializing now due to her inability to communicate adequately. She is either sleepy, because she must be heavily medicated due to violence and high anxiety, or exhibiting aggressive behavior. There is no longer a happy medium. This is the nature of dementia in some patients and certainly true for Mary. The only thing we know for sure that she truly enjoys is physical affection expressed to her so we make sure she gets plenty of it- hugs and kisses and words of affirmation.

We take her on outdoor wheelchair walks several times a day, when she is in a better mood, to get her some fresh air and a change of scenery outside. She also still enjoys sitting outside and watching the children play, but only for about 10 minutes at a time and then she gets anxious again.

My number one priority is her peace and comfort so there may be times when people come to visit that she is not coherent due to her medication needs. I do not want to be concerned with her being alert or awake when they come to visit if it means that it disturbs her peace of mind. Because of the great need to remain sedated, she no longer:
- is alert
- possesses the ability to speak clearly
- to be understood
- understand what is being said

It is better for her to be sedated right now than to be alert and undergo the torment she is in if I withhold the meds so she can try and communicate. Most visits occur while she is in bed because she feels safest and more comfortable there now.

This is taking some emotional adjusting for the family, but this is not my number one concern. I know that Mary is dying and she needs to depend on me to watch out for her comfort and put her needs above all else. Putting on her makeup and fixing her hair are not as important anymore and I have related this to the entire family.

She is in her bed most of the day now because she started "cocooning" last month. (This is when the dementia patient feels they must be surrounded by blankets and pillows to feel secure- kind of like a womb experience.) This calms her. After being in her GeriChair for about 15 minutes, she will begin to pound on it or shake it violently and yell out "mama!" or "Jones!"

She is still taking her clothes off so we keep her in the one-piece outfits so she cannot get to her diaper and shred it.

Sleeping Habits:

Mary never sleeps through the night anymore. We are still working with the nurses on adjusting her meds so she will sleep at night and awaken alert, but calm-it is a very delicate balance. We have her restrained in bed as well as in her chair so she will not be able to get up. She must be medicated most of the time so she cannot balance herself. She doesn't realize she cannot walk so we must protect her from herself.

Eating Habits:

At the present, Mary will eat about 20% of a normal sized meal. She is still on a normal diet but we supplement her lack of proper nutrition with the Nestles Instant Breakfast, 560 calories per can, 5 cans per day. We mix in chocolate, strawberry or butterscotch syrup to give her a variety.

She still likes BBQ and pinto beans, so we go to Bill Millers a couple times a week and get her a brisket plate. She also loves chicken fried steak and mashed potatoes with gravy. She will not eat much but she does have her favorites still. She will make it known by little groans of delight. Her favorite of all is chocolate candy with nuts.

Medications:

Mary is on liquid Lorazepam and Seroquel several times a day. These medications take the edge off of her severe agitation and violent behavior and make it possible to change and bathe her a little easier. I tried grinding up her pills and putting the powder in food but since she will hardly eat anymore, this doesn't work, however, she will drink down the liquid meds because they taste better. I wish they came in a chocolate flavor—we'd have it made! We still have to find the right nighttime med so she can relax and sleep through the night, without causing her to be groggy in the morning.

Physical:

I exercise Mary every day while she is sitting or lying down. I do ROM, or range of motion, exercises for her; I physically move her every joint and gently stretch out her muscles to avoid atrophy. This daily "work-out" is immediately followed by an entire body massage with Eucerin lotion for her dry skin. She no longer walks or is able to stand without assistance.

Mary's skin is in very good condition because of the numerous skin treatments and daily massages we give her. There is no skin breakdown.

She recently gained some weight. We believe this is due to our using great patience and determination in feeding her and getting the 5 cans into her daily. This does not mean she's getting better; just putting on a little weight due to the extra calories.

Bowel & Bladder Habits:

Mary is completely incontinent and her

bowels move every day at least once and most days 2-3 times. She tends to have bladder infections now and when she does, she gets more violent. Her nurse at the hospice works in concert with us to clear her up. We flush her system out with fluids and she goes on antibiotics. The bowel movements are very large. We change her between 7 & 9 times in a 24 hour period.

Mental & Emotional:

Mary has gotten increasingly violent over the past month. I realize that this is the progression of Alzheimer's disease. It takes 2-3 of us just to change her diaper because she fights so fiercely. We have to be very careful because she bites, kicks, pinches and punches. The less harmful; behaviors involve screaming, spitting and cursing. After we have her changed, we leave her alone for about 10 minutes and go back into her room and she is a different person. Her attention span lasts for about 10 seconds, which works to the benefit of all involved.

Bath time is extremely difficult. She never wants to take a bath. Anytime we have to disrobe her for any reason, she fights tooth and nail- literally! We all get a shower. We are still using the one piece, zip up outfits so she will not be able to take her diaper off and shred it. After repeatedly trying to tear the outfit, day after day, it does put a lot of wear and tear on them and eventually, they need to be replaced because the zippers get messed up or she tears different parts of them.

As you prescribed, we are using the vest restraint so she will not fall from the wheelchair and the bed.

Communication

I speak to her in very short sentences so she can remember the beginning and end of the sentence and hopefully have time to respond. The only questions I ask her are ones that require a yes or no response so we communicate very well this way. I make sure I get down to eye level with her and always smile while I talk to her or listen to what she is trying to communicate to me. She slurs most of her words and is difficult to understand, but we always take all the time she needs, to understand what she tries to say and this helps her avoid becoming frustrated. It also makes her feel valuable and loved.

She smiles at me all day long (unless I am changing her or giving her a bath!) and shows her appreciation of everything we do for her. She responds best to kisses, hugs and gentle and patient words of kindness and explanations, as do we all. She loves the kids and they give her a great deal of attention. She also tries hard to understand what they are saying to her. She is polite and courteous even in the dementia. We see no signs of depression at this time.

Requests

Since she has had ample time for the new meds to get into her system (3 weeks) and we have seen no change in the violence level or have they increased her ability to sleep at night, we ask you to change her meds.

You can either send this report to the doctor via email, snail mail or fax. Just be sure he receives it 2 days before the scheduled appointment so he has ample time to review it. Call to make sure the secretary receives it and then calls his nurse a day later to see if the doctor has read it.

HOSPITAL STAYS

How many times have you heard it said, "I do not like hospitals!"? One of the reasons we feel this way is because we associate a hospital with serious illness and death. Most of us do not know what's going on inside our own bodies and we may be afraid to find out.

If your LO has occasion to enter the hospital, you may have a chance to finally get a good night's sleep! Take advantage of the time in bed after you have him settled and are satisfied with the talk you have with the staff.

PLAN OF ACTION!

TIP # 1:

If this has not been an emergency admission, make your checklist for packing his things.

- Glasses, hearing aids, dentures and denture supplies
- Place all of his regular medications in a zip lock bag with a typed list showing the dosage, # of times taken daily and milligrams.

- Shampoo, conditioner, favorite lotion, toothbrush, brush/comb, razor
- Address book with phone numbers you might need
- Yours & his reading material
- Non-slip socks and slippers
- Light-weight robe
- Favorite pillows/blankets for you and him
- Snacks, gum, mints
- Legal paperwork such as living will, POA, guardianship

TIP # 2:

You will be asked if your LO has an advance directive. This means does he want to be revived and kept on life support if his heart stops. If he can speak for himself, let him answer the questions. If he cannot,
you should have already discussed this matter with him and if you have medical power of attorney (POA) for him, you can speak for him. If he wants to sign a directive in the hospital, this could be a good time to do so.

TIP # 3:

Some hospitals have suites which are wonderful if you plan to stay with him and can afford the upgrade cost. If not, see what the upgrade cost is for a private room and ask if they can provide a bed for you. If he is staying for only a night or two, you might want to stay at home and have another family member stay at the hospital.

TIP # 4:

Write down the names of

his nurses for all shifts and days he will be staying in the hospital. Write down the direct line to the nurse's station so you don't get the run around. Make sure all of the nurses have your contact information as well.

TIP # 5:

Pin the DON (Director of Nurses) down for the names of his doctors. You may think you know who his doctors are, but in many cases, there are doc's on the case you have never heard of. Get their contact information and titles and what the titles mean! You are entitled to this information, so don't be put off. Press in until you are satisfied. You may need to talk to these doctors. Also, find out what time each doctor makes his rounds and

who is scheduled to appear in your LO's room. This way, you can be there in that window of time.

TIP # 6:

Ask your LO's main hospital doctor if your LO qualifies for home health (if he isn't already on service with one). If so, the hospital social worker or discharge planner will get with you and discuss the number of times an aide can come over to help you bathe your LO and perform other grooming activities. Try and get the most visits and for the longest period of time allowed. You will need the help.

TIP # 7:

Stay on top of any new medications the hospital is giving your LO. There are many negative side effects with many medications these days. Also, after you have a list, check with your pharmacist about the possibility of them clashing with each other. It's a free service and you get quick results.

TIP # 8:

In regard to your relationship with the nurses and doctors, smile as you ask questions, watch your body and facial language and above all, show respect. Don't show your impatience or anger if he must wait for pain medication etc. Offer to help out with the care of your LO while you are there. They will appreciate that.

TIP # 9:

Keep an eye out for bedsores. Read our chapter in this book on "Skincare" for tips.

TIP # 10:

Do not be concerned about your LO becoming addicted to pain medication while in the hospital if he is in pain. All that really matters is his comfort and if that means he needs to be sedated to overcome the extreme pain that comes with surgery, so be it.

THE HOSPICE NURSE

If your LO is on hospice, he will be assigned a nurse who will come at least once a week and in between regularly scheduled visits when necessary. Her official title is "RN Case

Manager." The following is a list of the skills and services your hospice nurse provides: (she will…)

- Make a complete initial assessment of your LO's state of health.
- Present the hospice philosophy and the services provided by her agency.
- Explain your LO's rights and responsibilities.
- Assess wishes and expectations for everyone involved and talk over the resources available regarding his care.
- Provide volunteer support for you, your LO and/or your family.
- Teach you or your family how to physically care for your LO.
- Assess pain, pain management's effectiveness and other symptoms.
- Assess blood pressure and all other vital signs including pain.
- Provide comfort measures for pain and other symptom relief.
- Assess cardiovascular, pulmonary and respiratory status.
- Teach you symptom control and relief measures.
- Teach you how many liters of oxygen your LO needs.
- Teach you how to give medications to your LO, identify need for change, addition or other plan or dose adjustment.

- Teach effective oral care for your LO.
- Observe each week if there is the presence or signs of infection.
- Teach you and your family about realistic expectations of the disease process.
- Teach all involved the signs and symptoms of impending death.
- Teach you how to suction your LO safely.
- How to transfer your LO safely.
- Assess if choking and aspiration are going on and instruct you on what to do to help your LO.
- Teach you on safe eating measures.
- Assess mental status and sleep disturbances.
- Provide you and your family emotional support.
- Teach you how to turn your LO safely
- Teach you how to change the dressings for your LO's bed sores and how to watch for infection.
- Check for and remove impactions.
- Change catheter as needed.
- Teach you daily catheter care.
- Monitor bowel patterns.
- Counsel you regarding your LO's hydration, diet and nutrition.
- Explain the changes you should expect as your LO continues to decline.

She will confer with the hospice physician, develop a care plan in concert with the other hospice team members and order any medical equipment he needs.

She will take his vital signs; blood pressure, temperature, pulse and number of respirations and then record them on a report she will then leave a folder in his room. If he has any wounds, she will dress them. If he needs medication, she will order them and they will be delivered to your home that same day. She will closely follow his symptoms to see if there are any side effects to the medication and then make adjustments if need be.

If he is in pain, has fever, is having difficulty breathing or has any other medical need, she will contact the hospice doctor assigned to his case and receive instructions directly from him. She will also consult with you, give you care instructions and get your opinion on his care plan.

THE HOME HEALTH AIDE

If your LO is on home health, an aide will be assigned to come out 45 minutes to an hour, 3-5 times weekly. This will depend on the nurse's recommendation and the doctor's decision based on your LO's needs. This person is not a nurse but has been certified to do the following:

- Give your LO his bath (bed or tub).
- Clean his mouth and teeth and/or dentures.
- Apply lotion, moisture barrier ointment and powder.

- Change his clothes and diapers and his bedclothes.
- Shave him.
- Straighten up his room,
- Take out his trash and place his soiled laundry where you want for her to.
- Observe your LO's condition and report back to the team manager.
- Safely transfer your LO.
- Provide respite care.
- Prepare meals.
- Provide homemaker services.
- Provide comfort care.

She is *not* responsible for taking vitals or anything else that the nurse handles. She will report any change in your LO's condition in writing to the agency, and by phone if she feels the situation needs immediate attention.

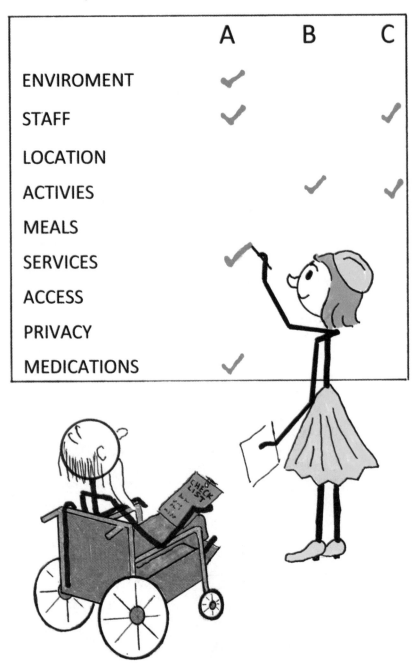

Did you ever have to make up your mind

-N-

NURSING
HOME
SELECTION
& ALTERNATE LIVING
ACCOMMODATIONS

THIS CHAPTER:

- **Nursing Home Checklist**
- **Independent Living Facilities**
- **Assisted Living Facilities**
- **Personal Care Homes**
- **End of Life Care**

NURSING HOME SELECTION

& ALTERNATE LIVING ACCOMMODATIONS

There are many forms of caregiving. Family members all over the world make the difficult decision everyday to place their LO in an alternate care facility. They visit their LO's at their new home on a daily basis; feeding them and making sure they receive the care and attention required.

Some spend many hours tending to caregiving chores at the nursing home. Then, they return home, get a good night's sleep and then they are back again the next day. If they are fortunate enough to have caring relatives, they take turns with the care.

There may come a time when you must turn the care of your LO over to someone else due to health reasons; your own.

This is why I decided to provide you with a checklist so you can make a wise and informed decision on a good nursing home.

NURSING HOME CHECKLIST

STEP 1:

To begin, let your fingers do the walking for a complete list of nursing homes in your area. The best way to find exactly what you're looking for in a facility is to "do your homework."

STEP 2:

Next, look at the following list of questions. Designate a spiral notebook for your phone interviews so they are easily referenced. Conduct a phone interview with the admissions director of each nursing home by asking these questions.

1) How long has your facility been in business?

2) How many residents do you care for at one time?

3) What is the staff to patient ratio?

4) How many people are employed there?

5) How many bedrooms do you have?

6) Do you provide transportation to and from doctor visits and is there any charge for this?

7) Is special assistance with bathing, dressing, and toileting provided?

8) What is a typical daily menu?

9) Do you know how to prepare food for special diets, such as diabetic, low sodium, or pureed diet? (This applies only if your LO is on a specific type of diet.)

10) How much experience do you have with hospice care?

11) What will you do if your LO has to get up at night?

12) Is there an exercise program available for the residents?

13) What kind of activities do the residents participate in?

14) Can my LO keep his own doctor?

15) Can my LO use his own furniture or do the rooms come furnished?

16) Can my LO bring his pet?

17) Can my parent have a phone in his room?

18) Can I come and have dinner with my LO occasionally?

19) What is the monthly fee?

20) Are there any other monthly costs?

Ask these questions during every phone interview with all nursing homes and then compare the answers. When talking on the phone with the managers, listen for and make note of any noises you hear in the background. Select your top three choices and then proceed to the next step.

(Do not feel obligated to make an appointment on the spot. Explain to the owners that you are just making phone calls at this point and that you will call back when you've made a decision.)

STEP 3:

Make your appointments to tour the nursing homes. When you arrive, pay close attention to the following details:

1) What kind of neighborhood is it in –
   Is it a place where you would feel your LO is safe?
2) How does the yard and grounds look —
   Is it clean and well-maintained?
3) Notice the smell when you walk in the building —
   Is there any smell of urine, mildew, etc.?
4) Does the house look cluttered or in good order?
5) Notice the number of staff that is visible.
6) Notice the appearance of the other residents —
   Do they look happy and well taken care of?

7) What were the residents doing when you arrived?

8) Ask to use the bathroom, and check it for cleanliness

9) How did the employees accept you when you came in — Were they courteous and accommodating, or did they seem hurried and indifferent?

10) Does the house feel like an inviting and cheerful environment?

11) Notice how the staff interacts with the residents.

12) Do the owners live on site?

13) Does the owner or person you spoke with on the phone look neat and clean?

14) Ask where the staff sleeps in proximity to the residents.

15) Ask how long the current residents have been living there.

16) Ask yourself if you would feel comfortable visiting your LO there.

17) Ask if the owner/manager has any objections to you contacting the families of their residents.

ALTERNATIVE LIVING ACCOMMODATIONS

INDEPENDENT LIVING FACILITIES

This is a retirement community for elderly adults who are self-sufficient. They have their own apartments, complete, with kitchenettes. Some of these facilities offer laundry service, have a beauty salon on site and a dining hall where their residents can dine if they so please. These apartments are ideal for the well-minded, wheelchair-bound, able-bodied and walker-prone seniors. They have no stairs to contend with, good lighting, extra wide doorways, ramps, sturdy furniture, and good security. They provide transportation to nearby stores and malls, church, meals and in-house activities. They can cost anywhere from $3500-$7000 per month on an average. They do not provide help with medications, bathing, toileting or cleaning of the residents' apartments.

ASSISTED LIVING FACILITIES

These places are classified by a variety of terms; personal care homes, board and care homes, adult homes, residential care homes. The residents who live in these homes need more help than an independent living community can provide. They can no longer cook or clean up after themselves or bathe unassisted. They may not be able to exercise sound judgment in decision making any longer.

Many things must be considered when selecting a facility of this type for your LO:

- Will your LO integrate with the other residents who live there?
- What kinds of residents are living there; able-minded, demented, mentally ill or retarded?
- Does your LO need a private room or if she wants a semi-private room, is one available?
- What is the resident to aide ratio?

Check out a good number of them and make sure that the one you finally settle on respects your LO's privacy and encourages him to remain active as long as is comfortably possible. Prices can range from $400.00-$3500.00 per month depending on services provided.

PERSONAL CARE HOMES

The good ones are a rare find, but they are out there. Private homes work hand-in-hand with home health and hospice agencies. Look in the yellow pages under "Home Health Agencies" and start calling. Ask for their social worker or patient care administrator and then ask for their list of private home providers.

This is a wonderfully comforting alternative to a more institutional setting. The caregiver doesn't necessarily have to have a nursing degree to care for your LO as long as she has practical experience, compassion and a heart for the elderly. While interviewing the candidates, you might consider using the following checklist.

THE VISION

Is the primary caregiver also the owner of the home? This particular type of care needs to be done by the person who originally had the vision for home care. Your LO needs a 24 hour commitment, seasoned with dedication and a wholesome pride in the work. The owner of the home is the person who came up with the idea to start a home for the elderly.

Many people buy or rent a home and hire a woman to live in and care for hospice patients. These people do not live in the same house as the patients; they have their own home elsewhere and this is mainly a business for them.

Because there is such a help turnover in the caregiving profession, if the owner does not live in the home your LO occupies, the constant need for training the new employee(s) could present a care problem.

When the owner lives and provides care in their own home, they are able to supervise the help, so you and your LO has at least one familiar personality to deal with regardless of the turnover.

You can rest easier when you go home because there is a consistent flow of heart-felt care day and night. All services performed for your LO are being continuously monitored. The owner/caregiver has their finger on the pulse of their home business at all times. This is not to say that there are exceptions, but difficult to find in an already extremely rare situation.

PRIVACY

Will your LO have a private room? This is very important for a bed-bound patient due to the need of privacy for friends, family, nurses, aides and clergy visiting. There are homes that even have an extra bed available for the family member who wants to sleep over at the end of their LO's life.

VISITING HOURS

What are the visiting hours? It is quite natural for a personal home to enforce visiting hours, however, if the nurse knows in advance that your LO has only a few days before they will be passing away, you need reassurance that the rules will be lifted, within reason, for friends and family to have the freedom to come and say goodbye.

RESTFUL ATMOSPHERE

Will the home environment be peaceful and quiet? There needs to be an environment in which your LO can relax quietly. It can be difficult for family/friends to visit if there is a noisy background. There can be disturbances from other residents and/or their visiting families. Children, dogs, loud television or radio cause distracting noise. You can always ask for references of those residents' families who are living there at the present and question them regarding such issues before making a decision.

NIGHTTIME RITUALS

Is the caregiver in the habit of getting up at night to:

- check on her residents,
- turn them when it is necessary
- change their diaper or toilet them?

END OF LIFE CARE

Do not fall into the trap of basing your final decision on the proximity of the home and allowing that factor to override the quality of the care provided there. All too often, families care more about how convenient it is for them (or friends) to visit, than the quality of the care. So what, if the home you pick is across town. If that home scored the highest on your list, make the sacrifice! Your LO's care, comfort, peace of mind and security far outweigh <u>your</u> convenience, doesn't it? It should!

If your LO is a hospice patient or has dementia, expect the monthly fee to be higher. There is much more care and attention to detail required when caring for someone who is dying or confused.

Just keep in mind that your money is there for THEM and their comfort, and that they should be made as comfortable as possible these last months or weeks of their lives. Keep it in proper perspective.

If they are in the final stages of life, it will not cost you or your family for very long. It will be over soon and you do not want to be feeling any guilt about saving a few dollars when you are attending their funeral. Many people spend more money on the funeral than they ever did for their LO's care.

You must consider all of this when making plans for someone to take care of them.

Also, if you just try to save money, disregarding the care (and you are truly able to afford better care), you may find that in a few months, that you got what you paid for and end up having to put them through an uncomfortable move anyway.

There are no shortcuts when you are dealing with someone's life. Take the time to make a quality decision, and when all is said and done, you will have peace and so will your LO.

As you interview each facility, be sure to take notes on:

1) the place itself
2) the people who work there
3) the owner (if possible)
4) the director (if it is a large facility)
5) the atmosphere
6) the number of years in existence
7) references
8) the number of terminally ill residents staying there
9) your own deep inner voice.

When you are finished with all interviews, crosscheck and compare your notes and then make the decision. If you go through all of these steps, you have a better chance of feeling peaceful about moving your LO.

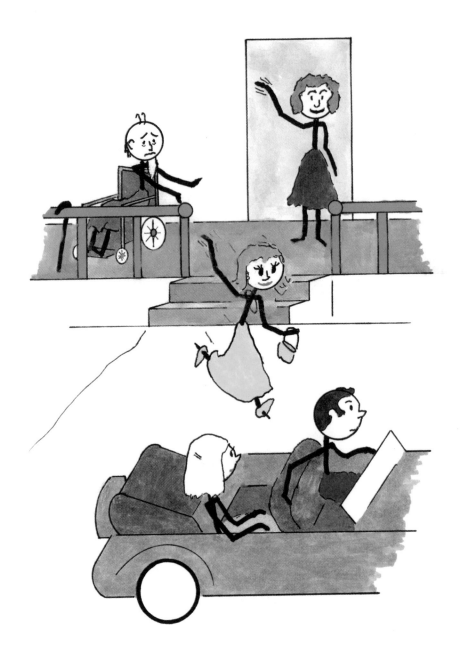

Friends

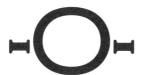

OUTSIDE
HELP

THIS CHAPTER:

- **Adult Day Care**
- **Church Senior Ministries**
- **Hiring & Managing**
- **Respite Care**
- **Senior Citizen Centers**
- **Trading with other Caregivers**
- **Volunteers**

OUTSIDE HELP

If you are working outside your home while simultaneously trying to provide the best care for your LO, you are going to need some help. You might as well face it right now; you cannot do it all alone.

Even if you are staying at home caring for your LO, you still need to go out and

get groceries, run to the cleaners, go out
with your spouse alone, go on vacation or
just go get your nails done. There are many
times you will need to leave him at home
while you go out so we have compiled some
ideas you may not have thought of in your
frenzy, trying to think of a way- some way-
to do it!

Adult Day Care

Turn to "Adult Day Care" in your phone book and start
calling the listings. Whether your LO is ambulatory, uses a
walker or is in a wheelchair, they can go to Day Care and give
you a much needed break to run your errands 5 days a week.
Your LO will be picked up by the facility between 8 & 9 a.m.
and drop him back off to your doorstep around 5, M-F.

Even if your LO has dementia, he will probably qualify for
their program. Just be sure to call all of the listings because the
prices vary.

In some states, Medicaid pays for these services, but if it
doesn't, ask if they have a sliding scale rate for you.

These centers will feed, exercise and provide company and
activities for your LO. He will start to look forward to going

each day. They have parties and promote friendship with others his own age.

Even if you must accompany him to "make" him try it, it's well worth the effort to get some relief.

CHURCH SENIOR MINISTRIES

Many churches have groups of individuals (what I call "Earth Angels") who will come to your house to sit with and entertain your LO so you can run errands or just go out for a while. They do not charge for this ministry usually.

If you are happy with a certain individual in their group, you might ask for their phone number to call when you are in a jam and tell them you can pay by the hour for sitting. This might be a blessing for both of you.

HIRING & MANAGING

If you hire a live-in helper/sitter, your caregiving life will become much easier. He/she can help with bathing, feeding, cooking, cleaning and keep your LO company.

The key is to keep trying different people out until you find the perfect match. You will have an avalanche of inquiries when you first put the ad in the paper, so keep track of the phone numbers and write down notes regarding each one you talk to or you will forget who is who.

Interview several of the top picks on the phone and then in person. Have one per day come over to observe them interact with your LO. At the end of the week, you'll either select one to return or start the process over again the following week. Don't be in a hurry to pick one.

PLAN OF ACTION!

TIP # 1:

The one you settle on should be friendly, diligent, kind, patient, aware of your LO's needs and be able to anticipate what he wants.

TIP # 2:

You can pay them by contract hire, which means that they file their own taxes. This way you avoid all the paperwork. We suggest paying $45.00-$50.00 per day (which means all the hours in a day

you need them) plus the extremely valuable room and board. This way, they receive cable, a bed to sleep in, their food, don't have to pay utilities and can save their cash each week! It's a great deal for all of you.

TIP # 3:

I also didn't pay any benefits like insurance etc. I was never a big company who could afford that and either can you.

TIP # 4:

I told them they had to be willing to work the weekends and have a day off during the week. I wanted to sleep late and go out on the weekends. You are the employer so make this easy on you- your help should not have the upper hand or make demands on you. Your attitude should be "I was looking for someone when I found you. Next!" I know this sounds cold but if you had been through what we have the past 18 years, you'd feel the same way.

TIP # 5:

Don't let your emotions rule you when selecting a helper. Don't feel sorry for them and think you must hire them or you really will be sorry later. If someone asks to bring their baby or

child to live-in too, say NO!!! You need help and there are many single women out there without children whose focus is you and your family- not theirs.

TIP # 6:

You don't want someone too young or they won't have the experience or maturity necessary to care for your LO. Many of the youth are eager to get the job but when it comes time for bathing or changing your LO, they are too embarrassed and will quit. All of the time you invested in training them has gone down the tube.

You don't want someone too old either because you don't need another patient to look out for; you need a helper who can stoop down, bend over and move faster than you can.

TIP # 7:

A good place for your new helper to sleep would be your LO's room. This can give you a sense of peace at night. If he is up most of the night, let your helper take the night shift and you take the days. Whatever works for you.

TIP # 8:

I never hired anyone that was married or was raising small children. Their mind would be on everyone but you and your LO. I hired single women, aged from 35-50 and they worked out nicely as long as they had some experience caring for elderly with diaper needs.

RESPITE CARE

Some nursing homes have respite services available. Respite means "break, breather, relief, let up." Does this sound good to you? Call around and check on their daily and weekend prices if you are in a jam and can't find a sitter. Tell your LO that this is only temporary and it will be a good break for both of you.

Make sure when you drop him off that you have a complete list of his meds, when and what to take, a contacts sheet that has his doctors listed and, of course, your cell phone and any other local relative's numbers in case of an emergency. If your LO has any peculiar habits. List them and the measures you take to deal with them In other words, don't leave them in the dark.

SENIOR CITIZEN CENTERS

Senior centers are scattered all over town, so investigate a few that are close to you and go visit by yourself first. You know what your LO likes, so pick one out and surprise him by taking him to lunch there. It's a great ice-breaker.

These centers are a place elderly people can go to socialize and eat together. They make new friends and can reminisce about days gone by with old photo albums and other mementos.

Many of them have a van that goes out and picks up the participants every morning and brings them back in the late afternoon.

TRADING WITH OTHER CAREGIVERS

If you want to meet other family caregivers going through what you are, join or at least visit a support group. There is a listing in the Sunday paper in most cities of all the support groups, so find the one that applies to your circumstances with your LO and go visit.

You'd be surprised how many caregivers need a break too and would be willing to watch your LO in exchange for their own day or weekend out. Start networking with others and see that there is relief to be found!

VOLUNTEERS

"Who in the world would actually volunteer to do all this work?" Well, call around to the churches and see if they have an elder's ministry. Also, if your LO is on hospice or home health, they have a volunteer's pool and they can send you a regular volunteer to come and sit with your LO while you tend to things outside the home.

With a little direction (like from our book) and creativity, you will see that your situation isn't hopeless if you get to work, make a plan and then put it into action. There are many people out there who are ready and willing to help you and it doesn't have to cost you an arm and a leg!

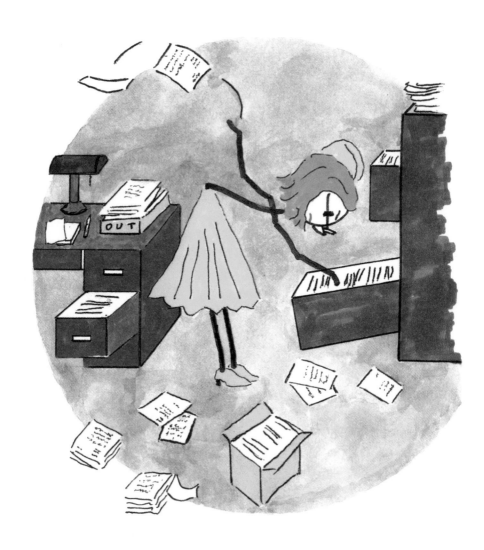

Ricky, Don't Lose
That Number!

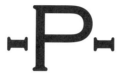

PAPERWORK

THIS CHAPTER:

- **Discovering & Locating Important Documents**
- **Your File System**

PAPERWORK

"B**aby boomers" or "the sandwich generation" — there are various labels used to describe this demographic group — and the facts speak for themselves.**

Census studies by the Administration on Aging, AARP and the National Alzheimer's Association have revealed that in the year 2000 there were 281,421,906 people living in the U.S. Of that number, 45,797,200 were over the age of 65. Within this population, 52% are mentally or physically handicapped and 33.4% are severely

disabled.

The most amazing statistic of all is that only 4.1% of our more than 45 million citizens over 65 are currently in nursing homes. This means that a staggering 43 million families are currently wrestling with what to do about finding appropriate care for their parents or are struggling to care for them themselves.

This is not a problem that will go away. The numbers of the aged in our population are climbing every year, and it is estimated that by the year 2030, there will be a staggering 85 million Americans over the age of 60! We still have a long way to go before we even peak.

If we take into consideration the fact that people are living longer (according to the Census Bureau, the average age at death in the year 2000 was 85), we can see that there are millions of Americans between the ages of 38 and 67 who are, of necessity, making decisions about arranging care for their elderly parents or grandparents.

Many of these caregivers have children of their own and the responsibilities of caring for them, both in the home and on the job; they want to help their parents, but they are simply overwhelmed. All too often, they suffer from a tremendous burden of guilt that keeps them from making important and sound decisions about their parents' care until it is too late — and their own health, careers or marriages are sacrificed in the meantime.

This is why I have included this vitally important chapter in my book. You don't need to be in the dark when it comes to your LO's state of affairs if you are his primary caregiver.

THE PLAN

If your LO is able to hold an intelligent conversation with you and has no communication problems, ask him about the following: (it would be wise to tape him audibly or better yet, to video tape this conversation)

If the LO is your parent, you've got to get past feeling like a child intruding on his privacy. Now is the time for action, and neither one of you have a choice. These things must be done. It's extremely important that you work on all of this before you get too busy caregiving and your LO is completely incapacitated to help you take care of his business.

The first step is to set aside some time when he is at his best and you will be alone with him, uninterrupted, for a few hours. It may be that you need to split up the time over several days, and they don't have to be consecutive.

Tell him that you need to discuss his paperwork. If he leans toward being paranoid about his money and doesn't usually share his private information with anyone, you need to address this first.

Explain to him that he trusts you with his care already, in fact, his very life depends on you. Tell him that if he doesn't share this information with you, you might not have the funds necessary to care for him in the future. You simply want to make sure he never has to go into a nursing home provided by the state. That you want to take care of him the rest of his life and then tell him the following:

"Isn't that what you want? You ask me why you should take the time to plan your care. It is imperative to prepare and organize all of your important paperwork ahead of time so that your exact wishes can be carried out, which will make it easier on all of us. If you don't help me with this and something were to suddenly happen to you, we'd all be lost. It would be extremely difficult to hold on emotionally while trying to make heads or tails of your bank information and insurance policies. I know you love me enough that you wouldn't want to put me through that!"

After he has agreed, it's time to get to work, so roll up your sleeves, get out a recorder or pen and paper and start taking notes.

DISCOVERING & LOCATING IMPORTANT DOCUMENTS

The following is a list of questions to go over with him:

1. Who is your family attorney? Where can I find his contact information?

2. Do you have a power of attorney? Who is it? I need his contact information. (If not, ask him to appoint you. If he agrees, make sure his attorney understands the type of POA you need to carry out his wishes and to have access

to all of his holdings for his future care. The POA expires at the time of his death. You need to have the POA notarized in the presence of two witnesses who do not have any interest in his affairs. The attorney will go into more detail regarding the rules. If he already has a POA and wants to keep this person as his POA, get with him to make sure he has all of the following information. If your LO wants to appoint a different POA, for example yourself, get with his attorney and tell him so. Then ask him the following questions:

3. Do you have a financial planner or an accountant? Where can I find his contact information?

4. Tell me where all of your bank accounts are. I need all of the passwords, balances and account numbers.

5. Do you have a current will; where is it and is it exactly the way you want it? (If he says he wants to update it, call his attorney and make an appointment for your LO to talk to him)

6. Where is your marriage certificate? (Ask this if your LO's spouse is still living. You will need this so you can help him/her file for benefits after your LO dies).

7. What current life insurance do you have? Where are the

policies? Have you been dealing with a particular agent? Where is the contact information located?

8. Do you have funeral insurance? Where do you keep the paperwork?

9. Do you have funeral arrangements made with a specific funeral home? Where is all of your paperwork located?

10. I need a list of all of your current credit cards and the passwords and balances on each.

11. Do you own any property that I don't know about? I need the details.

12. Do you have a safe deposit box? I need to know where it's located, the password and account number.

13. Do you have a pension or retirement plan with any of your former employers? Who are they and how do I contact them?

14. Do you have any CD's or IRA's? Who do you have them with?

15. I need you to help me list all of your assets and debts.

YOUR FILE SYSTEM

Place all of this information in a separate folder for future reference. This will take time to gather but you must have the information at your fingertips at any given time so get it done. Don't put it off. Depending on your LO's level of strength, it may take quite a few interviews, so start early.

If your LO has dementia or cannot communicate with you for this information, you need to initiate a search of his home and/or office. Enlist the help and legwork of your family. You may need to divide up the list among several people. Call a family meeting with a few of the more organized and diligent members. Schedule the next meeting with them (have them bring their weekly planners or calendars with them) before they leave. Tell them that you will all report on your findings at the next meeting.

This may sound like a lot of unnecessary work but if you've never been through it, you have no idea how important it is to get it done right. If you have been through it and not been this organized, then you will appreciate our attention to the small details.

Now that you know why and you feel convicted, let's talk about how to do it. The following is a check-list to help you record and legalize your LO's wishes and to organize all of his vital paperwork to keep in one place:

1) Go to an office supply store, like Mailboxes, Etc. or your

local post office and purchase a Living Will packet and help him fill it out according to the instructions. You can spend much more money if you prefer to enlist the help of your attorney, but it's really not necessary because the forms are very user friendly. Make a copy for your Power of Attorney and his attorney and get it to them. Make a folder marked "Living Will" and place the document in it.

2) If he has decided to invoke a DNR (Do Not Resuscitate) order and not enlist the aid of any artificial methods of keeping him alive, such as a breathing machine, etc., you can pick up the legal document at the places listed above. Follow the instructions, fill in the blanks, mark a folder "DNR" and place it inside.

3) In the event he becomes mentally or physically disabled and if he has sufficient finances available for private care, he needs to decide where he wants to be cared for, by you, a private nurse or agency, in a residential care home or specific nursing home. Write down his wishes and contact information, if applicable, and place the sheet in this folder. Make sure his POA and/or attorney has a copy of it and that he has expressed his wishes to all of your family members verbally, if he is able, to avoid future conflict in the event that he is no longer able to verbalize his choices.

4) Make a folder marked "Family Attorney," if he has one, and

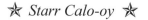

write down his contact information on it and place the page in this folder. (Make sure all information in the folders are legible; print clearly or type the information.)

5) Make a folder for his financial planner or accountant, if he has one, with contact information.

6) Do the same for his power of attorney. If you are his primary caregiver, this should be you. It should be one of his adult children that he trusts implicitly, a trusted friend in good health or another family member that he believes will carry out his wishes if he becomes incapacitated. Make sure the family attorney understands the type of POA he needs to carry out his wishes regarding his care, his personal finances and belongings and that his POA needs to have access to all of his holdings for his future care. The POA expires at the time of his death. You need to have the POA notarized in the presence of two witnesses who do not have any interest in his affairs. The attorney will go into more detail regarding the rules.

7) You need to make a folder marked "Bank Accounts." Designate a sheet for each bank account he has with all contact information, passwords, balances, account numbers and the person's name that he primarily deals with. Update these as needed.

8) If he has a current will, make a folder marked "My Current

Will" and place a copy of it in the folder. If he wants to update it, call his attorney and make an appointment to talk to him and get it done. Place another copy of the will with his POA in his safe deposit box, if he has one, but be sure to mention this on another piece of paper to include inside the folder.

9) If he is married and she is still living, place his marriage certificate in a folder so named. His spouse will need this if he passes away first so she can file for benefits.

10) Place his current health, life and funeral insurance policies in folders so named. If he has been dealing with a particular agent, write the name and all contact information on a sheet of paper and place it in the folder.

11) If he has funeral arrangements made with a specific funeral home make a folder and place all paperwork relating to it inside along with contact information.

12) Make a list of all of his current credit cards and the passwords and balances on each and place the list in a folder marked "Credit Card Information Sheet."

13) If he owns any property, write the details down and place the sheet in a folder marked "Property."

14) If he has a pension or retirement plan with any of his former employers, write down who are they and how they can be contacted. Make a folder marked "Retirement Plan" and place the paper in this folder.

15) If he has any CD's or IRA's, write down whom he has them with and any specific account numbers and passwords if applicable.

16) Make a list of all his assets and debts and place them in a folder marked appropriately.

Place all of the folders in a plastic, portable file box for future reference. This file box will contain his financial life, so you must make sure it's kept in a safe place. The attic is a great place if you have one and can get up there!

This will take time to gather but you and/or your family, POA and attorney must have the information at any given time, so get it done.

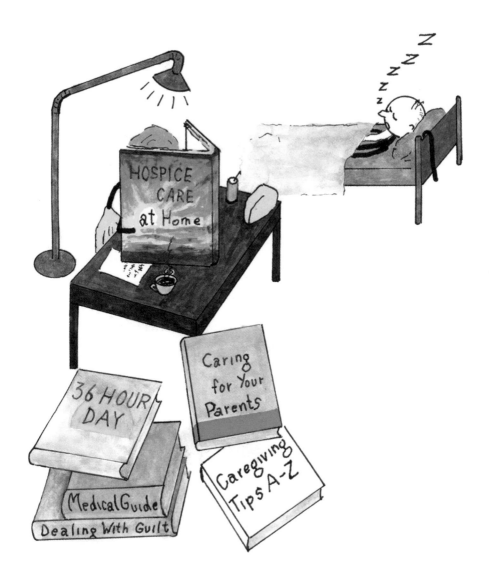

I Heard it Through the Grapevine

Q

QUESTIONS:
Frequently
Asked

QUESTIONS:
FREQUENTLY
ASKED

Question #1:

My mother has lived alone since my father died nine years ago. Now, she has AD and the doctor told us that she shouldn't live alone in the house any longer, but she will not leave. What can we do?

Answer:

It sounds to me that your mother is in the early stages of the disease and if so, you might try one of the following.

1) Tell your mother that her doctor thinks she needs some therapy and that the only place to get it, is at this place you've selected. If she feels that it is not a permanent move, she might be able to accept leaving her home. Assure her, that while she is gone, you will keep her lawn up, flowers watered, bring her the mail and take care of her pets. She

will be more apt to leave, if you set her mind at ease about the maintenance on her home while she is away. Tell her that the therapy lasts only one month to six weeks. Most of the time, dementia patients lose touch with space and time and are not able to judge accurately when a week has gone by, much less a month. Every day, when she asks, tell her she just moved in and it will be a month longer. After repeatedly saying this, day after day, she will come to accept it. When a month is up, don't tell her the month is over! This is the most merciful thing you can do for her. It is gentle. Don't feel that you are deceiving her for deception sake. Deception is a matter of the heart and is always conceived as a selfish act. This is not selfish.

2) Make up a coupon in the form of an invitation that says on it something like, "Surprise!! This coupon entitles you to a full month at our resort-like home. Manicures - Facials - daily massages - Pedicures - hairdresser - body therapy. It is all included!! Your family has already paid for this wonderful gift!!" Somewhere on the coupon, there needs to be the word, "Non-refundable". Place the coupon in a little box and wrap it up with a bow. Go visit her with several other family members, if possible. Tell her that you all have gotten together and have a surprise for her and then present her with the box. Make sure you are all smiling when you do. Celebrate with her. She will find it very difficult, even with dementia, to refuse such a gift from her LOs.

3) Ask her doctor to write a "prescription" for a one-month

stay.

4) Take her to see the doctor and ask him to tell her, in person, that he wants her to go to this place so she can get back on her feet again.

5) Ask her Pastor, Priest or Rabbi to come and talk to her. Arrange for other family members to be present when he comes.

6) Ask the new caregiver if she knows a social worker, if your mother does not have one available through a home health agency. Explain the situation to the social worker and see if she could help you by going to see your mother.

7) Ask a local fireman to come over and tell your mother the dangers for someone who has been diagnosed with this disease to live alone. Maybe he could also tell her some of the tragedies he has seen happen to those who did not listen to the advice of their physician and family.

Question #2:

Each time I go to visit my dad, he tries to prevent me from leaving. I feel so guilty, but I find myself going to see him less because I am running out of excuses to get away. What can I do?

Answer:

1) Before you go to visit, call the caregiver (if it is a small facility such as a personal care home) and let her know that if she has any business to discuss with you, to do it before your dad knows you are there. This way, he will feel that he has your undivided attention and that you only came to see him. Also, ask her to be available when you leave, to wait at the door (if he is ambulatory) and wave good-bye to you together from there. When you are ready to go, whether your Dad is bed-bound or ambulatory, kiss and hug him, say good-bye and walk out immediately. Do not respond to anything that he might say as you are leaving and do not turn around to look at him or wait for his approval. This might sound cruel but it is even more cruel and painful for both of you, to allow the goodbye to drag on. Reconcile yourself to realizing that you had a good visit and now it is over.

2) Get his favorite ice cream or candy and keep it out of sight until you are ready to leave. Just before you go, give it to your dad, love on him, say good-bye and leave immediately. A tasty treat may be all he needs to distract him so you can leave unnoticed.

3) Try visiting more often or less frequently to see what works for him better.

4) Find out when the next meal will be served before you

plan your visit that day. Arrive at the home in time to visit long enough before the meal. When it is served, leave.

Question #3:

My LO has Alzheimer's disease and has lost all equilibrium but I cannot keep her sitting down during the day. At night, she falls trying to get out of bed. How can I handle this dangerous behavior without being with her in the same room 24/7?

Answer:

Because self-compelled pacing and wandering is a common trait among dementia patients, when they get to the point that their equilibrium begins to diminish, they still have the compulsion. They do not realize that they will fall if they get up and there is nothing you can say to them that they can file away in their memory to make them understand the necessity to stay down. However, there are a few tips for safety's sake that might put your mind at ease. My methods might sound unconventional, but they have worked for many of the residents I have cared for in the past. Try these and see if any of them work for you.

1) Replace your traditional chairs for large beanbag chairs. They are much more difficult to get out of than a chair or sofa. Make sure that you place them out of reach of anything they could hold onto to aid them in their attempt to get up.

2) Put their mattress on the floor. This way, they do not have far to fall!

3) Ask your doctor to order a Geri-chair. This is a chair with a built-in tray that crosses their lap. They can eat on it and be kept sitting down when you cannot be in the same room with them, thereby helping them to avoid falling. Be sure that you get them up to move around or change postures frequently or they may develop sores and then you will have another problem to deal with.

Question #4:

I take care of my aunt who has dementia. She does many things that are very strange to me like taking her clothes off all day regardless of who is in the living room and she eats off of our plates at the dinner table. We cannot keep her out of the bathroom. She takes the clean towels out of the cabinet, wets and wrings them out and then hangs them all over the bathroom to dry. She probably uses a roll of toilet paper a day all by herself but she doesn't need it. It is just that she says she has to go but when she does, nothing happens, and she still uses the paper. The worst thing of all is that she will have a bowel movement in her disposable underwear, put her hand down in it, pull it out and play with it. It is a huge mess. She is quiet as a mouse when she does this. I am afraid to leave her sight. I want to keep her at home with me but I need some ideas on how to manage this odd behavior. How do I handle these particular problems?

Answer:

1) First of all, do not make the common mistake of thinking that she is doing any of this on purpose. Stop and think. Would you do any one of these, as you phrased it, "odd" things in your present state of mind? When she was your age, she would have never believed it if someone told her that in the future, she would be painting with her own feces. You are dealing with a brain damaged, elderly woman, not someone playing games to make your life miserable. What is imperative right now if you are serious about keeping her in your care, is to pray for strength, wisdom from God and creativity in dealing with these behaviors. If you aren't willing to do this, then by all means, find a good home for her with people who are called by God to care for her. Having said all of this, I have a few suggestions.

2) You can easily solve two problems in one step. Purchase a one-piece, zip up the back, long pant garment, (I use a fly-suit and I purchase them from Sears, in the men's department) and you can rest assured that she will not be taking her clothes off anymore or playing in her own bowel movements. She will not be able to figure out how to get it off if it is zipped up the back. Make sure that the material is not flimsy and that it has a good zipper on it and that it has long pant legs. One-piece shorts will never do. She would be still able to get her hands up inside her underwear. Just be sure to check her regularly to see if she has soiled her disposable underwear so you can help her change. If you will be consistent in having her wear this garment, after

about a month she will have "unlearned" this behavior and you will not have to put it on her anymore.

3) Make sure everyone seated at the table has extra food on their plates so that she can eat from their plates too. Are you surprised at my answer? Consider this, and please, do not be offended by my response. There will come a day that you will pray to the Lord, and have everyone you know praying also, for her appetite to increase. As the dementia progresses, they lose their appetites, their ability to swallow disappears and they have to have their foods pureed. Eventually, all they will tolerate is a high caloric liquid such as Ensure Plus by straw and ultimately, introduced into the side of the mouth by way of a large, plastic syringe. Then, at the end, you will not be able to give them any liquids at all, because everything you put into their mouth will go directly into their lungs because their esophagus will cease to function due to accelerated brain damage. So count your blessings right now, while you can. Sacrifice your sense of social etiquette for your LO and allow her to eat, whether it is off of your plate or out of the serving dish. At least she still has an appetite. Putting extra food on your plate and everyone else's is a small concession in the grand scheme of things, do not you think?

4) Another way to eliminate two of your problems at once is to put an eye and hook latch on the outside of your bathroom door, just high enough so she cannot reach it. Take her to the bathroom or ask her if she needs to go, every hour and

then accompany her. This way you can supervise her while she is in there. You tear off the appropriate amount of toilet paper you think is needed for her to use. Take the time to aide her and you will not have to monitor the open bathroom all day long and your clean, dry towels will stay put. Eventually, she will look to you to go to the bathroom and forget about staying in there all day as she is used to right now. Again, it will become an "unlearned behavior".

Question #5:

My uncle is in the latter stages of Parkinson's disease and has dementia and is staying with us. I cannot seem to get him to eat safely. He chokes on everything, even water. What can I do to help him?

Answer:

There are several liquid thickeners on the market. I personally use "Thickett" but there are others out there. You add this powder to whatever liquid you want to serve and by doing so, the patient is able to swallow much easier. Do not give him unblended foods. Make a list for yourself of soft foods he tolerates and put it on your fridge. Mashed potatoes that have no lumps, puddings (especially the high, caloric ones like Boost or Ensure), the soft insides of favorite pies, mashed beans, pureed spaghetti, ice cream (plain, of course; no nuts) or mac n'cheese.

This way, you can always have ideas at your fingertips to serve him. Give him small amounts, use a straw or a sipper cup

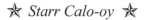
with the straw built in and stroke his throat for sensation sake as he swallows and be sure to verbally encourage and praise him for all his efforts and success.

Question #5:

Isn't there something that can be worn around the neck in case of an emergency?

Answer:

Yes. Acadian on Call. It's so easy to be safe with this user friendly system. All you do is wear the pendent around your neck, push the large button on it and you are connected with an operator who will help you immediately. Look it up online at www.acadianoncall.com or call Cindy Alleman 210-787-9699.

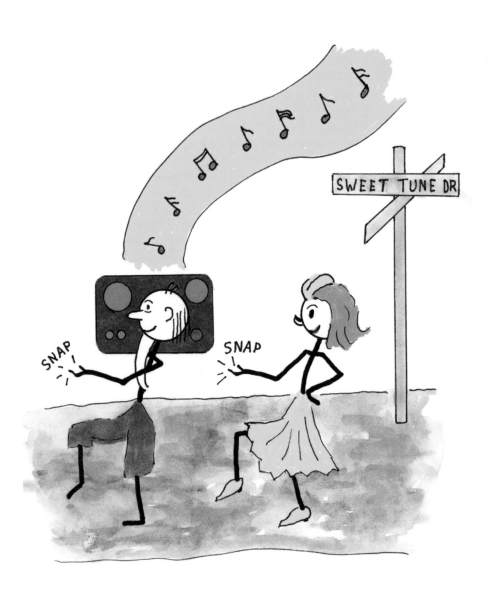

I've Got the Music in Me!

-R-

RECREATION, ACTIVITIES

THIS CHAPTER:

- Church
- DVD's & Music
- Family Parties
- Games
- Hobbies
- Outings

- Reading Material
- Sports
- Travel
- Tutors

RECREATION, ACTIVITIES

There is more to caregiving than grooming, making sure your LO eats well, is safe and his health needs are met. *I'm talking about having fun!*

We fill our children's lives with toys, sports, extra-curricular classes and parties out the kazoo. As we grow older, we crave bigger toys and the warmth of good friends and fellowship. We attend seminars and conventions and seem to be going somewhere or doing something all the time.

When we enter retirement, we may do some traveling if we are in good health, but for the most part, we move toward leading a more sedentary life. We lose touch with friends and co-workers. Our adult children are busy with their own friends, children and work.

Our bodies and minds begin winding down and we are on the outside looking in.

We no longer have the energy to participate and the younger generation is too busy to encourage us to use our wisdom and creativity so it goes dormant. Where did the fun go?

A caregiver has a responsibility to stimulate the minds of those in her care, but where does she start?

This chapter is chocked full of great tips you can take and run with immediately! If you stick with it, you will find something

that will get your LO's blood moving. He doesn't have to settle with being a couch potato the rest of his life and either do you. *Let's party!*

CHURCH

If your LO was accustomed to attending church all of his life and stopped when he could no longer drive or when he became too ill, he may be missing the spiritual support and fellowship he once enjoyed so much.

PLAN OF ACTION!

TIP # 1:
   Invite his pastor/rabbi etc. over to the house for lunch one afternoon. They can get reacquainted and become good friends, so find out the church schedule so he can start attending.

TIP # 2:
   If your LO is home bound, talk to the director of the senior's ministry at church and see if they can come visit regularly. Many of them bring their guitars and sing.

TIP # 3:
   If your LO used to sing in the choir and is still in relatively good health, encourage him to sing at home. After he has more

confidence, he might like to join the choir again.

<u>Tip # 4:</u>

If you aren't already, start praying with him before bedtime. It will cause joy and hope to well up in him again. By doing this, he won't feel out of place in church when he attends. At first, you need to make the first move and begin praying. Ask him if he would pray with you and soon, he will start initiating prayer himself.

DVD's & Music

Sensory activities are extremely stimulating and very important for the elderly because of their physical limitations.

Music can enrich your LO's life and bring back some great old memories. Use this avenue to get him talking and laughing again!

Old movies can do the same thing, so get out the popcorn and get ready to snuggle up to your LO!

Plan of Action!

<u>Tip # 1:</u>

My dad has a jillion albums from the 40's and 50's that he cherishes. I grew up listening to them all of my childhood. Maybe your LO has a collection too but it may be packed away in a box in the attic.

Get it out, dust it off and get an album to cd converter. This can be a great project for both of you to do together, depending on his ability right now, with the result being very rewarding.

TIP # 2:
Invite some of your older family members and his friends over for a retro get-together. Play their favorite music, bring out the photo albums, trophies, old mementos, and get the conversation going about the "good old days." Sit back and watch your LO come alive!

TIP # 3:
Put a small stereo system

in your LO's bedroom so he can listen to his music whenever he wants to.

TIP # 4:
Find out if he is interested in seeing any particular documentaries from the past and if he is, rent them from the video store.

TIP # 5:
Your local video store may carry DVD's of his old-time favorite music groups.

TIP # 6:
Ask him if he would enjoy taking a class on his favorite hobby by watching a DVD.

FAMILY PARTIES

As I mentioned earlier, families are going a mile a minute with their own lives. It's difficult for them to slow down and take the time to visit their elderly LO's. Because people are so goal oriented, setting a specific day each month to come visit will be more than feasible for everyone. If you act on these tips, you can virtually eliminate guilt caused by not visiting and give your LO something to look forward to every month.

Talk to your entire family about a monthly date everyone is agreed upon for a 2-3 hour family get-together at your home. It could be the 3rd Saturday of each month from 5-8, for example. Explain that this "party" will be held in your LO's honor. If they don't have time all month to come over and spend time with him, this would be a great solution!

PLAN OF ACTION!

TIP # 1:

Delegate! Assign different family members to bring the different dishes, chips & dip, sodas, tea etc. Make it easy- even if it's only sandwiches, the point is to let your LO see all of them together and be the center of attention.

TIP # 2:

Order a celebration cake for your LO. Have his name put on it and when you bring it out after all the main eating is done, make a big deal out of it. Have everyone clap for your LO and ask each member if they want to say something about or to him. They could tell him what he has meant to him during their life; what lessons he taught them that made a difference or tell a heartwarming story of a pleasant memory from the past that involved him.

TIP # 3:

Ask someone to videotape the party and another to go around taking still pictures. Post the previous months photos on a poster board for all to enjoy.

TIP # 4:

Make sure you fix up your LO for that day. Get him some new threads! Get his hair done. Make him feel special!

TIP # 5:

If you have a pool or barbeque pit in the back yard, make it a swimming

party. Don't do this if it's too hot or cold outside for your LO. The elderly are more sensitive to temperature. The grandchildren will love it and look forward to it too.

TIP # 6:

Tell all relatives to bring a little gift and wrap it up for your LO. It doesn't need to be expensive. Give them some suggestions for gifts.

TIP # 7:

If convenient and your LO is in good enough health to ride in a car and it's not too far, move the monthly parties from house to house.

TIP # 8:

Play your LO's favorite style of music.

TIP # 9:

In the midst of all the fun, don't forget to take him

to the bathroom or change his diaper. Make sure he is well hydrated, especially if the party is held outdoors.

TIP # 10:
Encourage all family members to bring old photo albums and videos/DVD's for all to enjoy.

GAMES

Games are a great source of entertainment regardless of your age. You can sit down, laugh, fellowship and really get to know each other while playing. We have always had games going at home and we have learned a lot about each other by playing regularly.

When I was growing up, dad taught us how to strategize by playing checkers and the value of the dollar by playing Monopoly.

What games did you grow up playing? Bring them back into your life now and you won't regret it. This is good for all of you; not only your LO. If your family has not indulged in games as a lifestyle in the past, start a new family trend. You will all have fun.

PLAN OF ACTION!

TIP # 1:
Learn how to play "42" if you don't already know how. The instructions are in every box of dominoes. It takes 4 players and is very addicting!

This game was a regular family tradition when I was growing up and we have continued it. Dad comes over and plays with Bob, Charles and I and we play for hours. It will keep you and your LO sharp.

You can set a certain day of the week to play. Serve dry snacks.

TIP # 2:

Did your LO used to play pool? If you or your relatives have a pool table and your LO is able to get around, ask him to shoot a few games with you.

TIP # 3:

Table games are great fun. What kind of card games did he play in his younger years? Was it poker? If so, get a game going and invite some friends or family over to play. It may have been Spades or Fish. Whatever it was, break open the box and get to playing!

Checkers are entertaining too. If there isn't a Cracker Barrel restaurant close to you, go to www.crackerbarrel.com online and order their "3 in one Jumbo Checkers." They are only $11.99 and so much fun to play with.

TIP # 4:

Anyone for Bingo? Find a bingo hall in your town, take your LO, if he is able, and enjoy. Make sure you don't get so involved in your own cards that you neglect helping him with his.

HOBBIES

It may have been a long time since your LO has had a hobby he enjoyed, but ask him if he would introduce you to this part of his past. He may have an old stamp or coin collection tucked away in a box somewhere that he would really enjoy dusting off and tinkering with again.

PLAN OF ACTION!

TIP # 1:

If your LO is on home health service, talk to the social worker about getting him occupational therapy. The therapist will work with him 2-3 times a week with his favorite hobby.

TIP # 2:

Look online or in the Sunday paper for the hobby club in his genre and take him to one to see if he could get interested in it again.

TIP # 3:

If he used to love gardening but you know that would be too exerting for the state of his health now, get him to start a potted herb garden. He could keep that on his windowsill or the back porch. Keep him in supplies to sustain his interest.

TIP # 4:

If he had any kind of collections in progress when he got sick, help him resume them.

OUTINGS

Can you spell "cabin fever?" We all need to get out of the house every now and then.

Don't look for your LO to exhibit the same symptoms as you do before you take him out. He might simply retreat to his room and pull the covers over his head. If you see him do that, and he's not ill, get him out of the house and take him to a place you know he has enjoyed in the past.

If he is reluctant, tell him that you need an escort and that it's for you-not him.

PLAN OF ACTION!

TIP # 1:

If you have small children or grandchildren and he can be depended on to keep a close eye on them, drop him and the kids off at McDonalds to eat and play. He might enjoy watching them laugh and tumble around.

If he needs supervision too, either go with him or delegate someone to sit with him while you both watch the kids.

Ask him if he is willing to help you out by doing this for you. Most of the time, he won't refuse and will leap at the opportunity to be helpful.

TIP # 2:

Plan a certain day each week to take him out to his favorite restaurant. Let him choose.

If there are other willing

family members, ask them if one of them could plan a specific day in the week each month to take him. Learn to delegate!

TIP # 3:

Take him to the movie theatre. Get your tickets online to make it easier on you. Go during the week, during the day so you don't have to wrestle with the crowds.

TIP # 4:

Take him to a play or a concert.

TIP # 5:

If the weather is just right, go to the zoo and takes lots of pictures.

TIP # 6:

Tour your city with him but only for a few hours at a time.

TIP # 7:

Make a list of the places he used to go with his spouse and start going. Allow him to reminisce.

READING MATERIAL

Ah, the lost art of reading. Our entertainment is so visual these days that less and less people are into books. However, the elderly grew up reading so encourage him by using these tips.

PLAN OF ACTION!

TIP # 1:

If your LO's eyesight permits, take him to the bookstore and get him excited about reading again.

TIP # 2:

Designate a 30-minute time slot for you to curl up with a book in the living room and read. Each of you read your own literature or take turns reading to each other.

TIP # 3 :

Take him on a trip to your local library branch and encourage him to select books from his preferred genre.

TIP # 4:

If he likes reading magazines and he has a favorite, order a

subscription. He will look forward each month to receiving it in the mail.

TIP # 5:

If your LO cannot read due to poor eyesight, get him a few books on tape. You can pick them up at Barnes & Noble. They have a wide variety in every genre from which to choose.

TIP # 6:

If he is computer savvy, even a little bit, pull up a list of online books on the web. As long as he can be taught to scroll down, he will be able to read it. He can also make the print as large as he wants for easier reading.

TIP # 7:

When we were caregiving, our small children, still in elementary school, would read to our residents every evening. It was a blessing to both of them. If your LO is still well-minded and likes children, maybe they could help you by working with the children while they do their homework.

TIP # 8:

Have your LO's eyes checked twice a year and their glasses updated so they can enjoy life.

SPORTS

Watching sports on television with the guys is as American as stars, stripes, and homemade apple pie! Boys are brought up playing ball of all kinds.

Just as women identify with cooking, cleaning and child rearing, men find part of their identity in getting together with the guys and their sons to watch football, basketball and hockey.

PLAN OF ACTION!

TIP # 1:

If he is able-bodied and has the desire, take him "out to the ball game." Make it a family event and let him invite

TIP # 2:

If your LO has been watching a particular sport on television most of his life, make the effort to keep an eye on the TV guide to know when it comes on. If it's If your LO has been watching a particular sport on television most of his life, make the effort to keep an eye on the TV guide to know when it comes on. If he watches a specific team, turn it on.

TIP # 3:

Our family is into basketball- big time! We live in San Antonio, Texas so we never miss the San Antonio Spurs games. They play 2-3 times a week and all of our friends and family know they can come over to watch the games, eat and fellowship. We have an open door policy.

If he is a big fan, open your doors to friends and family and have them bring the food. It can be a lot of fun for your LO and perk him right up! Try it a few times to see how your family feels.

TRAVEL

Mother was sick and unable to travel with daddy for the last 8 years of her life except one trip they took with my sister, Debi, and her family. They had always planned to travel when they retired but it didn't work out that way.

Since mother passed away, daddy has taken several big trips with my sister and had a marvelous time seeing sights that he and mother had planned.

If your LO can travel, consult him about where he has always wanted to go and then take him if he is able to go.

PLAN OF ACTION!

TIP # 1:

Take your LO in to the doctor for a full check-up and get his okay for him to travel. If you are going by plane, ask the doctor if your LO is up to it. If he will be in the car for extended periods, ask him about that. Some elderly have circulatory problems and tend to swell in their ankles and feet.

TIP # 2:

Be sure to order all of his meds in advance of the planned trip so you don't run out. Also, take allergy and cough medicine, ibuprofen, Band-Aids, etc. Keep them handy.

TIP # 3:

If you will be traveling by car, take an ice chest and stock it with plenty of juices and water. You don't want him to get dehydrated.

Take individually packaged nuts, cheese sticks, yogurt, carob covered raisins or nuts etc. for snacking.

TIP # 4:

If he sleeps with a certain pillow, be sure to bring it along. If he requires blood sugar testing, make sure you have plenty of supplies. If you take his blood pressure daily, bring the equipment.

TIP # 5:

Purchase long, vinyl-covered lap bibs. They will keep you clean and are great for everyone in the car!

TIP # 6:

Try to keep to the same bedtime ritual and time as

you do at home. Make sure you give him his meds at the same time every day as you do at home.

TIP # 7:

Don't let him get too hot or cold. The elderly are extremely sensitive to temperature changes and he needs you to watch out for him.

Keep in mind that you and your family move at a different pace than he does, so don't wear him out. Let him go at his own pace.

You don't have to see everything if it's at his expense. It's not worth it.

TIP # 8:

Take lots of photos and videotape of him. You will cherish these one day

TUTORS

It's never too late to learn! There is an old saying, "Stay green." As soon as we get ripe, we rot and fall off the tree. Tutors aren't only for our children.

Is there a certain subject your LO is interested in learning more about but is homebound so cannot attend the classes? Get him a tutor that will come to your home and teach him.

Plan of Action!

Tip # 1:

Call the colleges and find out if there are students who are enrolled in a work program where they get credit for coming out to tutor your LO in the area he is interested in. They do this as volunteers for part of their grade score.

Tip # 2:

Call your nearby school district office and ask them for a list of their tutors by subject category. Interview them over the phone. If a tutor only has one day a week to come and you find that your LO wants more than that, get 2 tutors!

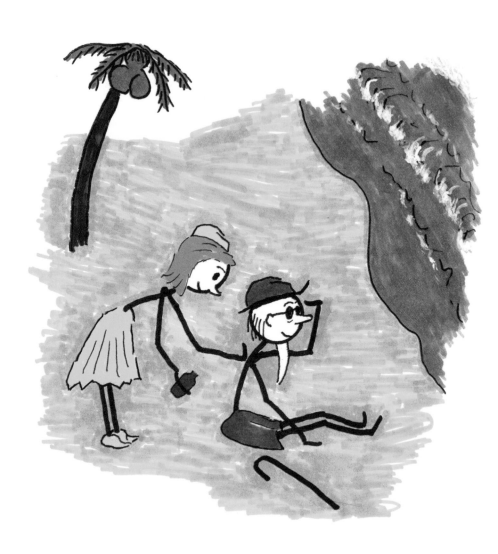

I've Got You Under My Skin

˙S˙

SKIN CARE

THIS CHAPTER:

- **Pressure Sores**
- **Dry Skin**
- **Bruising**

SKIN CARE

If your LO sits most of the day or becomes bed-bound and his brain fails to send messages to the skin cells to repair or replace themselves, it can result in pressure sores or bed sores.

As his primary caregiver, it's up to you to protect his skin from painful and life-threatening conditions.

The following tips may help you prevent sores from occurring to your LO and if he

already has them, may help to get rid of them.

PRESSURE SORES

A pressure sore is an open wound on the skin, which occurs because of prolonged and constant body weight in one specific area of the body. In severe cases, it can become infected and the skin breaks down, in some cases, to the point of rotting away to the bone beneath.

Pressure sores can happen when a person is confined, due to medical reasons, to a chair or a bed. When the person gets close to death, it doesn't matter how often you turn them, they can still appear because the skin cells are no longer receiving, or acting on, the repair messages that the brain is sending.

Below are listed some preventative measures you can take to prevent this very painful condition:

1. Check his mattress to make sure it's not too hard. Hospital beds come with a non-removable plastic cover on their mattress that becomes hardened over time. A gel mattress or alternating air pressure mattress can be very beneficial when placed on the bed of a bed-bound patient, if he can no longer shift his position on his bed. If he has home health care or is on hospice, the nurse will come over, assess the situation and ask the doctor to place the order. Unless your LO has an open bedsore, he won't qualify for a gel-pad or air-pressure

mattress under Medicare guidelines, even if he is on hospice service. If you want one, you may have to buy it from a medical equipment and supply store.

2. If your LO does have an open wound, call his nurse or doctor to report it and ask them to order the gel mattress for him.

3. Sheepskin heel and elbow protectors should be worn to prevent pressure sores. Your home health agency, hospice agency or local pharmacy will have these in stock. You can also request from his doctor or buy for yourself some sheepskin heel protectors from the pharmacy or medical supply store. Keep his feet clean and if his skin breaks open anywhere on his body, call his doctor or the hospice agency immediately.

4. Turn your LO over (if he can't move around by himself) every 2-4 hours.

5. There may come a time when you need to turn him every 2-3 hours from side to back to side again. When you turn him on his side, place pillows between his knees, legs and feet (so that they do not touch), 1-2 propped up behind his back and if in an electric hospital bed, bring the head down electrically. Don't bring it down completely, but almost flat so that he isn't cramped.

6. If the breakdown is on his heels, place a pillow under his ankles so that his feet hang off and the heels don't touch any surface. When on his back, be sure to elevate his head to keep the pressure off his tailbone.

7. If he is bed-bound and cannot turn himself, massage his entire body with massage lotion or baby oil twice to three times daily to stimulate circulation.

8. Keep his skin clean and dry. Gently rub out red areas with a moisture barrier ointment when first observed.

9. Call the doctor or nurse as soon as you notice any redness developing. This is a sign that sores are brewing beneath the surface. It is of the utmost importance that you rub out the red areas before they turn color. When red changes to dark purple or dark blue, this is just before the skin blisters and then breaks open. If left untreated it can develop an infection, become toxic, rot away and can eventually result in a more painful death.

10. Skin breakdown can occur in some very surprising places for example, if your LO wears a catheter for his bladder, be very careful to protect him from his lying on his own tubing. It can cause a pressure sore in a matter of hours. If he is on oxygen and wears a nasal canula with over the ear tubing or a

mask with thin, elastic straps that are worn over the top of the ears, skin breakdown can occur very rapidly.

11. If his head rests on the bars of his hospital bed, for even an hour without being moved, it can result in skin breakdown.

12. A neat little tip I discovered when I tended to a boo-boo on one of my children one day, is to brush 5-10 coats of Liquid Band-Aid, over the affected area, allowing each coat to dry before applying the next. The area is protected because the pressure is removed and the skin has an opportunity to rest and heal itself. You can use this behind and over his outer ears to avoid sores from forming from the oxygen tubing.

You need to protect your LO in many ways and it may seem like a lot of work, but it is worth doing when you consider the alternative. If your LO develops pressure sores, there will be much more pain and the increased work load to go with it.

DRY SKIN

As we get older, our skin loses the ability to re-hydrate itself when it gets dry. The natural oils, which are abundant when we are children, become scarce.

Dry skin turns into itchy skin which causes people to scratch off any oil that is there, leading to even drier skin.

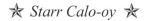

Listed on the next page are a few suggestions you might try if your LO has this problem.

1. Do not bathe your LO any more than 3 times a week.
2. Do not make the water too hot otherwise, you risk drying the skin out more than it already is.
3. Use a moisturizing rather than a deodorant soap.
4. Keep the oil out of the tub for safety reasons, but pour it on and rub it in outside of the bathroom after the bath.
5. Use cotton clothing.
6. Cut some fresh Aloe Vera directly from the plant. Peel it, boil it with a little water and then when it is cool, apply it to the dry skin. Do this twice daily.
7. Use a very soft washcloth to bathe him. If you can get a cloth baby diaper, that would be best.
8. Eucerin lotion (found in most drugstores) is great for dry, itchy skin. Be generous in applying it. It will not leave your LO's skin oily either,
9. Water consumption will begin to re-hydrate his skin as well as flush toxins from his body.
10. If he will not stop scratching, use cortisone cream or calamine lotion.
11. Caffeine will cause the itching to worsen besides not being good for him anyway.
12. If it doesn't let up, take him to a dermatologist or his doctor and have him examined.

BRUISING

As we age, we tend to bruise much easier. Our skin gets thinner and we do not heal as quickly as we once did. Bruising, simply defined, is bleeding under the skin and the more translucent it is, the darker the bruise.

You may have noticed that when your LO has had an injection, a large, purple bruise appears the next day. When we are younger and have the same injection, you see little or no sign of it.

Bruising is normal for the elderly but if this is a new thing for your LO, have it checked out by his doctor. It could mean he is starting to have clotting problems.

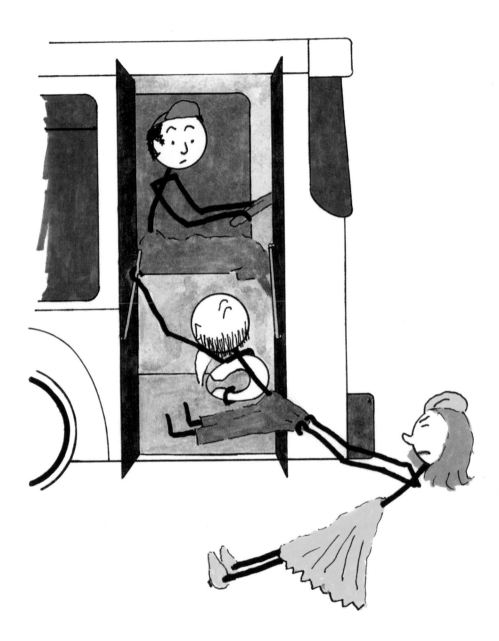

Ticket to Ride

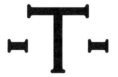

TRANSPORTATION

THIS CHAPTER:

- **How to Transfer the Non-ambulatory**
- **Public Elderly Transportation Door-to-Door**

Transportation

If the thought of moving your LO terrifies you because you are afraid you might both fall down, we have a few ideas for you.

There may be occasion for you to send your LO to therapy or a doctor's appointment because you are unable to take him yourself. If so, the tips in this chapter might help you.

HOW TO TRANSFER THE NON-AMBULATORY

People think that weight has something to do with their ability to lift and move someone but if they do it correctly, it doesn't.

My dad taught me how to lift correctly when I was young and I have used this method all my life. I had to go to a chiropractor several years ago and he x-rayed my back. He was surprised to find that I had the spine of a 20 year old with a full inch of cartilage between each vertebra. That was after 18 years of caregiving; lifting patients from bed to wheelchair, wheelchair to toilet, wheelchair to shower etc.

If you haphazardly lift or move your LO, over the years you will develop back problems.

FROM BED TO WHEELCHAIR:

- Remove the leg lifts from the wheelchair. Place the wheelchair at a slight angle, close to the bed. Put the brakes on.

- Pull your LO up on his bed as high as he can go. Electrically or by hand crank, bring the bed up to a sitting position.

- Lower the bed as far as it will go down to the floor.

- With one hand holding his neck and one arm under the crook of his knees, slowly spin him around to a sitting position, facing the wheelchair.

- Place your arms around him, interlocking your fingers at the small of his back.

- Place your knee between his legs and in one quick, safe movement, lift and pivot him into the chair by riding him on your knee.

FROM WHEELCHAIR INTO SHOWER
OR ONTO TOILET:

- Before you placed him into the wheelchair for his shower, you should have undressed him and covered him up with a towel. If he wears a diaper, this should have been removed as well. Nothing should hinder the transfer once you begin.

- If going to the toilet, bring down his pants and remove them completely. You don't need to be wrestling with clothing.

- Remove the leg lifts from the wheelchair once it is facing the tub. Put the brakes on.

- Place your arms around him, interlocking your fingers at the small of his back.

- Place your knee between his legs and in one quick, safe movement, lift and pivot him onto his shower bench by riding him on your knee.

- Swing his legs into the tub and keep him covered.

PUBLIC ELDERLY TRANSPORTATION DOOR-TO-DOOR

Call your local Agency on Aging or Alzheimer Association to get a complete list of vans, buses and private drivers who make pick-up and deliveries. Some are free resources and some charge for their services.

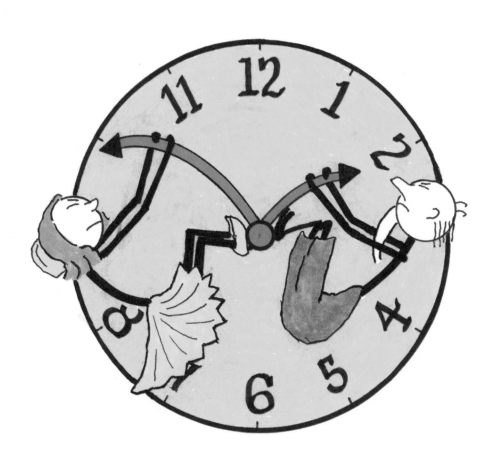

It's Too Late

-U-

UNRESOLVED
CONFLICT

THIS CHAPTER:

- **Then & Now**
- **The Blame Shame Game**
- **How to Forgive & Grow Up**
- **Marie's Story**

Unresolved Conflict

I walked into Omar's room just in time to stop his daughter's hand from coming down on his head. I caught her by the wrist.

I said firmly, "We don't do that in our home."

Omar was 91 years old, our very first patient and was in last stage of Alzheimer's disease.

Her name was Cindy and she tried to explain, "You don't understand. He put my entire family through hell while I was growing up. He was mean when he was drunk and he drank all the time. He beat my mom and all of us kids. He would slap us across the room for nothing.

We all hated him and now, he puts us through having to take care of him? He doesn't deserve your care. You are too good to him. He should be suffering right now.

Now, after 45 years, I finally have the courage to tell him how he hurt me, and he doesn't even understand what I'm saying. It's just not fair!"

I can't begin to count all of the adult children whose LO's we cared for over the years that expressed the same feelings. They didn't forgive their LO's when they

were well-minded, so they suffered from a lack of closure when dementia came suddenly. This is one example of unresolved conflict.

This is not an easy issue to address and there are no easy solutions, but we will attempt to help you with a few tips in this chapter.

Like everything else, it will take some work and introspection on your part, but in the end, it will be worth it. Peace always is.

Then & Now

Would you carry a 25 pound bag of smelly garbage around with you everywhere you went, every day, for your entire adult life? Would you open it and pour it on your floor each evening and then gather it all back up as you headed out the door for work or to the store the next day?

If you are actively remembering and dwelling on the faults, sins and transgressions of your LO every day of your life, that's exactly what you are doing.

Your LO is a completely different person than he was as you were growing up and so are you. Did you ever think of that?

I don't care what he did or didn't do right when he was younger. That was then; this is now. We all change. We all make mistakes. We all grow.

Learn to live in the present, not the past. What will your children say when they stand over your grave? What will they remember most about you?

When it's you in the bed, dementia or not, how will they care for you? With resentment of the past or will they look at you as you are then; helpless and at their mercy?

Remember, you are sowing every moment of your life. You either sow seeds of life or seeds of death. What does your crop look like right now?

Regardless of their ages, you are teaching your children how to treat you by the way you are treating your LO right now. If you show unconditional love and have patience with your LO, others will have the same for you when you need it the most.

THE BLAME & SHAME GAME

"Shame on you!" This is one of the most toxic and lasting curses we could ever put on our little ones. We don't even know the extent of the damage we cause when we try to put shame on others.

Here is another familiar phrase: "Dysfunctional family." Almost every criminal that gets caught, blames their actions on their parents and the family they came from instead of taking personal responsibility themselves.

We blame other people all of our lives for everything wrong with us. We want justice for those who wrong us and we want mercy and grace from those *we* wrong!

Now, we take full credit for our virtues, desirable qualities, strengths and goodness in spite of our terrible upbringing.

I am not being cynical or stereotyping the human race here but many, many people are like this. If this does not apply to you and you give credit to your LO for your turning out as good as you did and you have no unresolved conflict in your life, skip this chapter!

However, if this sounds at all like you or someone you know who is struggling with these emotions, read on to discover a few ways to find peace while caring for your LO with dementia.

How to Forgive & Grow Up!

So, you want to forgive your LO, but you don't know how. Many people carry their past with them for thirty, forty, fifty or more years, allowing it to distort and pervert the rest of their lives. They do not realize that they are seeing their loved one as they were, not as they are now.

Before, he was strong, had the ability and inclination,

maybe, to be manipulative, deceitful, cruel and unfair. Now that he has dementia, he simply doesn't have the mental capacity to do those things anymore.

It may be difficult for you to change your perception of him because you have spent most of your life on equal and sometimes competitive ground, matching wits or trying to please him.

When your LO became demented, your roles changed and he became the "cared for", dependent, frail, helpless and confused. He no longer had the strength or mental capacity to be mean anymore. This change is practically impossible to wrap your brain around, especially if you both have had a lifetime of ill feelings and harsh words between you.

Let me make a few suggestions that might help you resolve this inner turmoil.

PLAN OF ACTION!

TIP # 1:

Unforgiveness will hurt *you*. It's like drinking poison and expecting your LO to die. It doesn't work like that. Forgiveness is a decision- not a feeling. You decide to forgive and then your heart begins to line up with your decision. It takes time- it's not instant- it took many years of layer upon layer of hurts to form this crusty shell of protection. If you are consistent about resolving to forgive him, it will happen. One day you'll wake up and realize you are free! Jesus laid down His life for your sins. The least you can do is forgive your LO his sins against you.

TIP # 2:

There are many people who feel as you do about wanting this nightmare to be over. As hard as it is, investigate a support group in your area for families of AD, such as the Alzheimer's Association. Find out when they meet and attend the meetings. Listen to their stories so that you can see that you are not alone.

It is only after they get together and end the isolation that they begin to come to terms with this dreaded disease of the mind. Your LO does not necessarily have to be diagnosed with AD in order for you to attend. As long as he has a type of dementia and you are having difficulty coping, you can go to share with the others.

TIP # 3:

Make some calls to different hospices, settle on one and then go meet with their chaplain and social worker. They are more than familiar with the depression, unforgiveness due to unresolved conflict and fear you are experiencing. You may find that your LO is a prime candidate for their hospice program and if so, they will support you all the way through the journey you are all going through.

TIP # 4:

Accept the role changes that exist now. At one time, your parent cared for you and nurtured you; now it's your turn to see to it that they are cared for. Realize that things will never go back to the way they once were when you looked to them for guidance, strength and advice. You have to be the one to make the decisions now and there is no room or time left for bitterness or resentment. This is your shining moment to give your parent the honor and help that God commanded you to.

The Word says that when you do that things will go well for you (and this includes your own physical, mental and emotional well being) and you will live long upon the earth.

TIP # 5:

Make an appointment with your pastor and get some Godly counseling and direction. You may need an outside opinion on how you are seeing things. Don't let your pride get in the way. Your loved one needs you mentally and physically healthy, especially now.

TIP # 6:

Take time to get away to be with your spouse and children or if you are single, with other siblings or friends. Go somewhere with different surroundings and a change of scenery and when you do, don't feel guilty about enjoying yourself. When you return home, you will feel a renewed strength and see things in a new and proper light. You need a fresh perspective.

I would truly be remiss if I didn't include the following true story about what obedience to God and forgiveness did for several people, a few years ago. This is another amazing example of God's love and perfect timing in bringing about peace, reconciliation and showing us that it's NEVER "too late."

MARIE'S STORY

Marie was a very responsible young woman. Although she was forty-three years old, she was still single and living at home caring for her parents. Her dad had early stage Parkinson's disease and her mother had been diagnosed with AD.

She worked all day at the bank and would come straight home to help her dad with mothers care. Her other siblings helped as they could, but the brunt of the care fell on her shoulders. She longed to be married and have children but her responsibility and loyalty for her family was always more important to her.

Kay, Marie's older sister, was diagnosed with breast cancer in December of 1996, so both sisters joined a prayer chain at their church. Marie was assigned to intercede for a seventeen year old boy dying of AIDS, so she tacked his picture up on her bedroom wall and prayed daily for him and his family for a month, but he died in January.

As she cut the obituary out of the paper, she noticed that another boy, Jeff, died the same day in a car accident, so she cut that one out too and put them both up on her wall to pray for their families. She prayed that if Jeff's family didn't know the Lord, that God would send someone to minister to them in their grief and lead them into the kingdom so they could find peace.

About that same time, one of Marie's best friends, Dawn, was diagnosed with an inoperable brain tumor. Every day, without fail, as soon as Marie got off from work, she would go to Dawn's house to cook for her family and clean up the house and then go home to care for her own parents. This was truly a labor of love and the Lord gave her the strength and ability to accomplish all of this work with joy.

For several years, Dawn had been sharing with Marie about situation with Mary, her supervisor at work. This woman was manipulative and cruel to all of the workers under her authority and had singled Dawn out specifically. Dawn's reaction was to pray for her and to try to do what she was told without incident.

One morning, while Dawn's husband, Andrew, was at the store and she was alone, Mary came to see her. The door was open so she let herself in.

She began, "I know you must be surprised to see me today, but I've come for two reasons."

"First, I wanted to tell you how sorry I am for the way I've treated you all these years and ask your forgiveness."

With tears in her eyes, Dawn responded, "I have forgiven you all along. I never held anything you've ever said or done to me against you. On the contrary Mary, I've been praying for you all this time. But you said there are two reasons?"

Between her sobs, Mary answered, "I've never told you this before, but I have great respect for you. In all the time I've known you, you've never lashed out at me when I've been unfair to you. I know that you are a Christian and that you're close to God."

She continued, "I've been told that you aren't going to live much longer, so I've come to ask a favor of you. My son died last month after we had an argument, so I was hoping that you'd tell him something for me when you see him."

Dawn's heart was filled with compassion as she said, "I'd be glad to do that for you. What do you want me to tell him Mary?"

"Tell him I was proud of him and I'm sorry for all the things I said at the end. Tell him I love him and that I should have shown him how much he meant to me but I was prideful and angry. Tell him I said he was a good son." Dawn had never seen Mary more genuine and broken.

As weak as she was, Dawn motioned for her to come over to the bed and these two women embraced. There was reconciliation, forgiveness and blissful closure. Andrew came home just as Mary was leaving and Dawn told him everything that had happened. That night, Dawn went on to be with the Lord.

After the funeral, a reception was held at Dawn and Andrew's home. Mary and her husband attended. While Andrew and Marie were talking, he pointed Mary and her husband out to her and related the story Dawn told him the night she died. Marie, moved with compassion, reached out to them and went over to introduce herself. All three of them went into one of the empty rooms and Marie ministered to them and led them to the Lord.

When they were about to leave, they mentioned their son's name; Jeff. It was then that Marie realized that he was the same young man, the stranger, whose obituary she had cut out the month before and put on her wall. Little did she know at the time, that the Christian she prayed for to come and minister to this strangers' family, would end up being *her*!

Marie continued going over to care for Andrew and his two children in the evenings and weekends. One day, Andrew gave Marie Dawn's ring and told her that Dawn wanted her to have it. They bonded through the love they shared for Dawn. Several months later, Andrew proposed to Marie and she accepted.

They continued caring for Marie's parents and her mother went on to join Dawn a few years ago. Her father is now in the last stages of Parkinson's disease, living at home, under the loving care of Andrew, Marie and her siblings who lend a hand when they are able.

She still lives at home, works at the bank and now has the family she always dreamed of and they are still serving the Lord today in Colorado. She has been my best friend since we were 12 years old.

Through Marie's obedience and Dawn's forgiveness, a hard heart was softened and closure was achieved as unresolved conflict was settled once and for all.

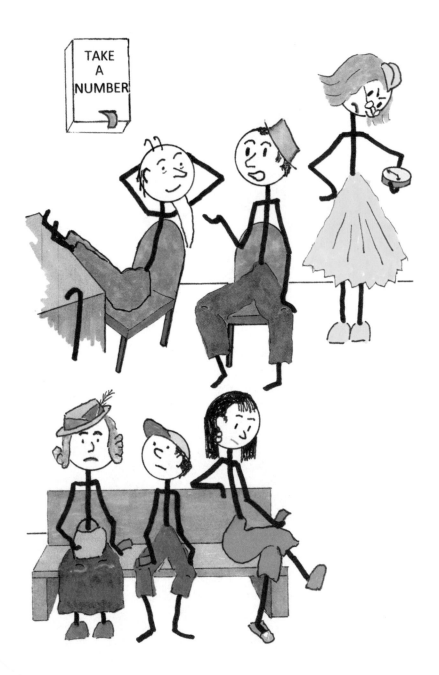

Got to Get You into My Life

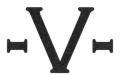

VISITATIONS

THIS CHAPTER:

- **Family & Friends Visitations**

VISITATIONS

There are some very important things you need to know about visitations that will occur in your home, so I am going to speak very frankly about them with you in this chapter.

Everything I share with you is from my own personal experience, so I hope you or your family won't be offended with my frankness. It is never my intention to offend anyone, but to enlighten people and avoid misunderstanding before it happens.

Having said that, please realize that because you are the family caregiver and are providing 24/7 care in your home for your LO, everybody (including you) needs to respect your right to privacy. Many home caregivers feel that if they care for a family member, they must have an open door policy and that all visitors have a right to come whenever they please. Most of the time, it's their own relatives that impose or force their will and desires onto the caregiver.

I cannot say it emphatically enough; you are responsible for maintaining control of your own home. You not only owe it to yourself, but to your spouse and children still living at home.

You have already sacrificed so much of your life to provide loving care for your LO. No one else in your entire family stepped up to the plate because of their career or family demands (as if you didn't have a life too).

Most of the time, relatives who have refused to care for their LOs are the first to criticize and the last to help when the caregiver really needs a break.

These attitudes are very common so know you aren't alone. Below are some tips to help you survive the parade of visitors that will inevitably beat a path to your door! Implement them to keep your sanity.

PLAN OF ACTION!

TIP # 1:

In order to keep peace, set the boundaries. Decide on which visiting hours you and your family can comfortably live with and then enforce them. Once you start making exceptions, you will get the rest of the family mad at you when you don't do it for them and if you do, you might as well throw the rules out the window.

You have very good reasons for your visiting

hours and don't have to spend all of your time explaining yourself and the decisions you have made to anyone. Stick to your proverbial guns! No means no!

TIP # 2:

If your LO is on hospice, you will have to make sure he gets his rest, so visiting hours are essential. For guidelines, solicit the counsel of his nurse and then inform the family verbally and in writing. Ask the nurse to sign it to show the family that this is not your idea alone, but the best thing for your LO. Give everyone a written copy of the days and hours your LO will be available to visit. Be sure and include a disclaimer that states the hours are subject to change depending on:

1. the previous night's sleep
2. behavioral difficulties during the day of the planned visit
3. something that comes up unexpectedly in your own family

Also, mention in the disclaimer that your priority must be the welfare and comfort of your LO, not the family's convenience.

This may sound harsh but if you have already been a caregiver for some time now, you will completely identify and agree and if you are just starting out, you will soon understand what I am talking about.

TIP # 3:

Regular family visitors

can be useful to you by helping your LO at mealtime by feeding them, if they need assistance and the visitor does not distract him from eating. This can be good for both parties involved.

When a family member or a friend can do something to help your LO in any way, they regain some sense of control in their life. They can't control your LO's illness and feel helpless, standing by, watching him deteriorate, so this can be therapeutic for the visitor. Don't ever feel you are imposing by asking for help.

TIP # 4:

You need to take time to visit your LO also. We get so caught up in the day-to-day, hands-on caregiving work, that we don't sit down and talk, listen, play, read, eat or even touch our LO's in an affectionate manner. It's not that we are cold or uncaring- there is just so much work to do.

If your LO likes coffee in the morning, sit with him and have a cup also. Talk to him like you don't live there! It will take some practice, but you can do it and make him very happy. Look at the world and your house from his viewpoint. He sees you moving at the speed of light all day. Relationships- that's what will matter the most when he is gone. Your morning coffee talks will remain sweet memories- not the laundry!

TIP # 5:

If your LO becomes

agitated each time after seeing a particular visitor, it's up to you to talk to that person and curb the visits for a while. You are your LO's defender and protector, so if he is unable to speak up for himself for whatever reason and you notice a change in his behavior, it's your responsibility to handle it for him.

If he is well-minded, try talking to him about your observations and allow him to open up. Let him know you are there for him and that if he doesn't want someone to come over, he doesn't have to confront that person himself- you will and very nicely.

TIP # 6:

Please be mindful of your LO's privacy and maintain his dignity. Have visitors leave the room during diaper changes and other private procedures. Don't use the words "diapers", "bibs" or any other word in front of others that would cause him embarrassment. Be aware of your actions and words whether others are around or not. Show this elder respect and servant hood rather than any form of domination or supremacy.

TIP # 7:

Many times during the years of caring for people in our home, when visitors would come over during mealtime, their LO would get so excited that they stopped eating. I had to change the time they ate so no one would be present to distract them. It's well worth the effort because the alternative can be a weight loss they cannot afford.

Sometimes they stop eating because they get embarrassed by the way they have to eat because of denture or other mouth problems, so again, try to remain hypersensitive about what is happening right before your eyes. Most of the time, they just won't tell you the problem- you have to second guess all the time.

TIP # 8:

It would seem that visiting should come naturally, right? Actually, most people do not know how to visit effectively and there have been some good books written on the subject so I won't attempt to cover all mistakes people make, but will cover a few of

them.

If your LO is hard of hearing, don't shout, but speak clearly while looking at them at eye level, a little louder than you normally would. Then, adjust your volume slowly, until you have reached the correct level for them.

Always try to smile while you speak unless the subject doesn't lend itself to glee!

Reassuring touches, on the arm or hand-holding usually communicate sincerity. Express your love and concern for them by using genuine facial expressions.

Watch your body language as you listen to them. If your legs or arms are crossed, this communicates a closed mind and spirit, even if you are more comfortable doing so. Point your body in their direction as you converse with them.

TIP # 9:

Invariably, there will come a time when your LO deteriorates to the point in their health that they don't want you to fool with their hair, make-up or fancy clothing. They will want what is practical and comfortable as opposed to what is more appealing to the eye.

Do not put them through the ringer getting them ready for visits if they feel this way- even if they haven't expressed this to you because they may not be able to.

Many well-meaning family members want your LO "fixed up" because it makes *them* feel better. The most important thing is to do what makes your *LO* feel better.

TIP # 10:

Do not prop them up in a wheelchair if they cannot sit up by themselves just to satisfy family and friends who stop by to visit. If he cannot sit up alone, leave him in his bed. Please don't make the huge, common mistake most caregivers make in trying to gain the approval of onlookers at the expense of the weak or ill elder you are caring for!

I cannot tell you how many family members insisted I "walk" their LO's, not knowing that the following day they would pass away. I never did- I was the caregiver and knew my patient could not walk or even sit and really didn't care what everyone thought about me. All that mattered was the comfort of my patient and whether he could voice it or not, I knew

God was smiling on the conviction I had.

Don't make your LO perform "tricks" for anyone!

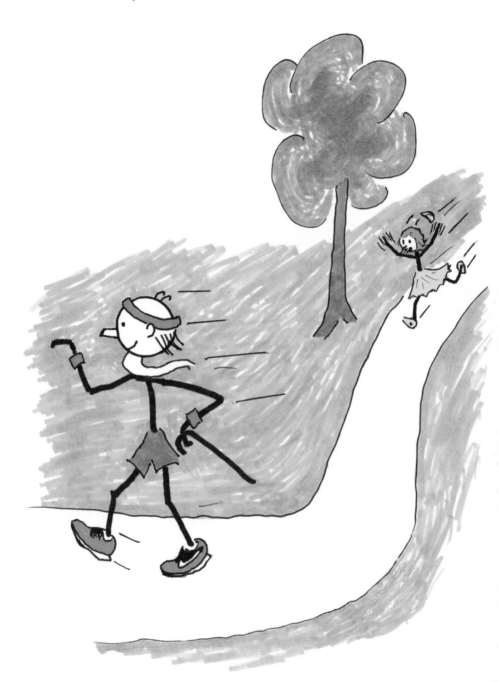

Walk This Way

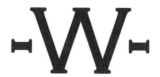

WALKING

THIS CHAPTER:

- **Shoes & Apparel**
- **Hydration**

WALKING

This is not an extensive chapter on exercise. We will be discussing how to help your LO to prevent atrophy (deterioration of the muscles).

The elderly are fragile, so we must be very careful when it comes to leading them through any kind of exerting activity.

Many elderly people seem to think that exercise is optional instead of mandatory. *Wrong!*

Everyone knows how good walking is for their health. It's all over the media's. Your job is going to be to sell your LO on the benefits. We will share a few of them with you.

Knowing *how* to walk your LO is key to their receiving the maximum benefit.

If he is ambulatory, walking can improve his heart, reaction response, range of motion and his awareness. A daily walk can ward off depression, anxiety and promotes a better mood.

Some of the nice things about walking is that regardless of the weather, he can experience a good walk indoors. I wouldn't put him on a treadmill, but he could easily walk around inside your house if it's raining outside.

Also, you don't need to buy any special equipment for walking. If you walk him outdoors, you could choose a scenic area like the zoo or botanical gardens in your city.

Practicing walking on a regular basis, will keep him ambulatory longer than if he didn't walk.

Watch him walk. Does he naturally shuffle? Get him to pick up his feet for safety reasons. Is he standing tall or does he walk stooped over? After you make a secret evaluation, have a talk with him and practice walking correctly.

Time to walk the walk!

SHOES & APPAREL
PLAN OF ACTION!

TIP #1:

Buy your LO a pair of walking shoes from a sports shoe and apparel store instead of a department store. They will know to fit him for a size larger than his normal shoe size- if they don't do this on their own, leave the store, go home. Make a few phone calls and find a store that knows this. They will have the type of footwear you need for him.

TIP #2:

Be aware of the weather he will be walking in. Layer his clothing if it is a little cool so he can dispense with articles of clothing as he gets warmer.

TIP #3:

Buy him light, cotton socks so his feet can breathe.

To begin regular fitness walking, the only equipment you will need is a pair of well-cushioned, supportive shoes - trainers, specialist walking shoes or other suitable footwear. Many shoe manufacturers now routinely build in cushioning support in their shoes, even smart business shoes made by companies like Ecco, Rockport, Clarks, etc. You might also want to invest in a pair of cushioned walking socks to give further protection to your feet.

HYDRATION

During physical activity, the body loses water primarily through sweat, even in cold weather or in water. The body has several mechanisms to protect itself from the negative effects of dehydration, but thirst does not occur until the person is already dehydrated!

The following are a few guidelines to follow while your LO struts his stuff!

Dehydration means your body does not have as much water

and fluids as it should have. Dehydration can be caused by losing too much fluid, not drinking enough water or fluids, or both. Vomiting, excessive exercise and diarrhea are common causes. Even if your LO doesn't have a walking routine, it is important for him to drink plenty of water. Listed below are some of the more common symptoms of dehydration:

- Dry or sticky mouth
- Low or no urine output; concentrated urine appears dark yellow
- Not producing tears
- Sunken eyes
- Lethargic or comatose (with severe dehydration)

PLAN OF ACTION!

TIP #1:

As soon as we experience thirst, we are already dehydrated. If you plan to walk with your LO, start hydrating him early by making sure he drinks 1-2 cups of water that morning.

TIP #2:

Have him drink 1-2 cups of fluid 30 minutes before walking.

TIP #3:

Have him drink ½ - 1 cup of liquid for every 15 minutes of walking. I know this seems like a lot of water, but you'd be surprised how much water we lose with even a little exertion.

Tip #4:

It is better to have frequent, small amounts of fluid, rather than trying to force large amounts of fluid on him at one time. Drinking too much fluid at once can bring on vomiting.

Tip #5:

If you get serious about his walking daily, go to the pharmacy and stock up on electrolyte solutions or freezer pops.

Tip #6:

Avoid giving him sport drinks. These usually contain a lot of sugar and can completely alter his bowel movements.

Tip #7:

If he refuses water because he doesn't like it, try giving him Crystal Lite. It contains no sugar, sodium, calories, caffeine etc. They come in a wide variety of flavors and are delicious! The main idea here is to find what works to keep him hydrated.

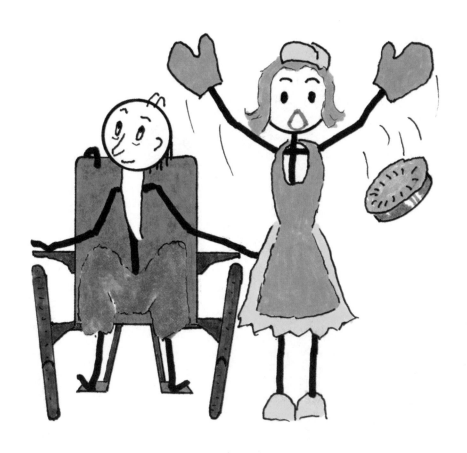

Good Golly, Miss Molly!

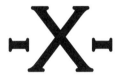

X-RATED

THIS CHAPTER:

- **Inappropriate Sexual Advances**
- **Masturbation**
- **Stripping**

X-RATED

What comes to your mind when you read these words: public stripping, masturbation, unwanted sexual advances?

When a well-minded individual displays these behaviors, they are often locked up and need a lawyer to defend them!

However, when a person with dementia does these things, we need to reach out to them in compassion, not recoil from them in disgust.

Confused people sometimes have an absence of social awareness. They forget where they are or that it is proper to remain dressed when in the presence of others.

Just because they are elderly and have dementia doesn't mean they no longer have sexual urges or the ability to become aroused.

They do not realize that masturbating out in the open is wrong. It feels good to them and that is all they know. How you handle this will be the mark of either a true caring caregiver or an immature and judgmental bully. Let me give you a few pointers.

STRIPPING

You walk into the room and you see your LO naked as a jay bird. What do you do?

Wrong reaction:

You get angry and embarrassed and start yelling at them. You tell them something like "What in the world do you think you're doing? What can you be thinking? Are you crazy? Put your clothes back on this instant!" You start jerking them around.

Their response is one of total bewilderment and they may start crying or getting angry at you. They are fearful and may even become embarrassed realizing they have no clothes on. They may even think in their confusion that you have removed their clothes and fear you and start making accusations which in turn makes you angrier. You lose control.

Now, if you think that by behaving in this manner you will prevent future episodes you are WRONG! All you have done is to get both of you very upset.

When you calm down and regain your composure, your LO will all but have forgotten what happened and just be angry with you or worse, afraid of you, but you will be ashamed of your behavior, realizing that they did not even know what they were doing. There is a better way.

Correct response:

As soon as you see them, you do not say a word. You go to the closet and get a robe for them. You return to the room and cover them as you begin to dress other body parts. You make casual conversation, never referring to the fact that they have just taken all of their clothes off. If they want to fight you or argue, tell them very slowly and softly that "We need to get ready to go outside to go for a walk." If it is raining, tell them anyway.

When they are dressed, take them outside or into another room and get them busy stacking books, folding laundry, counting pennies or give them a sweet treat to eat. In other words, distract them.

PLAN OF ACTION!

TIP # 1:

If they keep taking their clothes off, buy a one-piece jump suit that zips up in front. It is an outfit that is a top and pants all in one. Take the collar off, make a V-neck and put it on them backwards. They will not be able to unzip it. Not very fashionable but it works. We have found that when they have worn these for at least 3 weeks, they no longer remember the **unwanted** behavior anymore and we can return to their normal attire.

TIP # 2:

If you are in a public place, you should be able to catch your LO long before he has completely disrobed.

All you do is distract him gently, with a smile, and if that doesn't work, get him to the car and take him home.

MASTURBATION

If you discover your LO masturbating in a room other than their bedroom or bathroom, there is a way to handle the situation so that they will not get upset. Here are a few do's and do nots.

1. <u>Do not</u> become obviously alarmed, displaying anger, shame or superiority.
2. <u>Do not</u> touch him in any way to make him stop. This could result in his becoming combative or even violent with you.
3. <u>Do not</u> talk down to him regarding what you have just witnessed.
4. <u>Do</u> gently lead him into a private room.
5. <u>Do</u> try and distract him with ice cream or his favorite sweet treat or another activity.
6. <u>Do</u> tell him that you want to take him outside for a walk and then proceed to re-dress him. Be sure you are smiling and speaking softly and that your tone is gentle.

INAPPROPRIATE
SEXUAL ADVANCES

It is rare, but your LO may make sexual advances such as groping or verbal innuendos to you or others. Again, they do not know what they are doing. This is not an excuse. You are not going to be able to get anything "through their head" by getting angry and yelling at them. In most cases they are beyond "learning" new behavior.

Sometimes, a man may behave in a sexual way toward his daughter. In his mind, she may look like her mother, his wife when they were much younger. If you are that daughter, it does no good to repeatedly tell him that you are his daughter, not his wife. Hold his hands gently and distract him from the subject.

Above all, love him and keep telling yourself that your dad needs your understanding.

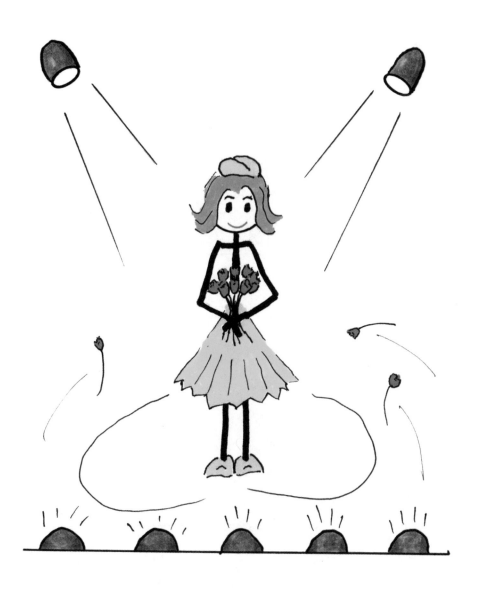

Shining Star

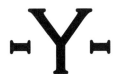

YOU! THE CAREGIVER

THIS CHAPTER:

- **The Taffy Trap**
- **Caregiver Burn-out**
- **Depression & Isolation**
- **Caregiver Illness & Death**

YOU! THE CAREGIVER

For eighteen years as a caregiver, I was the first one up in the morning and the last one to bed at night. Can you identify? Of course you can!

Your entire life is consumed with caregiving topics, techniques, questions and answers. You live, breathe, eat and sleep caregiving.

You may feel you are losing your own

identity because you don't go where you used to go, don't do the things you used to do and don't see the friends you used to see before caring for your LO. But you *are* more than a caregiver and we hope to give you some things to ponder, realize and apply in this chapter.

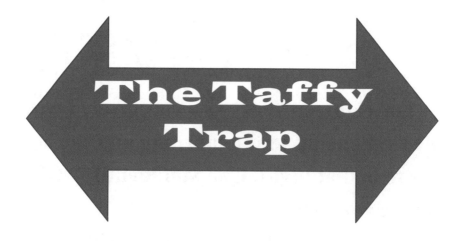

What is "The Taffy Trap"? Well, caregivers these days are pulled in many different directions, even to the point of feeling that they have lost their identity. Sound familiar?

It's true that since the beginning of time, caregivers have had to wear many hats in their everyday life, but it's only been since our men came back from World War 2 that they enlarged the borders of their job description.

Before the war, most women stayed at home and took care of the household responsibilities exclusively. When the war came, they had to take over their husbands jobs so that their men could go off to war and fight for our nation.

Before this point in history, their husbands took care of the finances, the yard, the household repairs, taking little Johnny to basketball practice. Enter: modern day caregivers and "The Taffy Trap."

Later, when their men came home from the war, women had the added responsibility of caring for him as well. They didn't want to give up their careers that they had worked so hard to develop. This is when America's divorce rate began to escalate. The roles were reversed with, seemingly, no solution in sight.

Men's attitude, justifiably so, was "If you want to work, fine, as long as you continue to fulfill your household duties." Naturally, husbands wanted their wives to care for them, the children and the home but this caused a great deal of stress and strife in the American household.

It wasn't until the last few decades that America has become a 2 income family. The reason for this was that new technology was developed to meet the escalating workforce. There was a need for new inventions to make life easier for the working family. Along with the new and improved gadgets, came a more expensive lifestyle.

Daycare for tots became increasingly expensive, which led to longer work hours and more education, which led to less

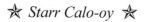

time, spent at home. Now it is no longer a preference for mom and dad to work outside the home- it's a necessity.

Being a baby boomer is just as taxing on our women. If you have teenagers, you have another huge list of added responsibilities as well as the stress that comes with it! Just keeping your sanity and remaining even-tempered is a chore in itself. Women are still suffering today from being pulled into many directions at once. Multi-tasking is second nature to the modern woman. A woman must have coined that phrase!

Let us take you through a typical day in the life of an American caregiving woman who **also** works outside the home. We'll call her Mary:

1. Mary wakes up in the morning before anyone else does. She showers, dresses, gets her make-up on for the day, puts on her "Valet" **(valet role)** hat, and helps her husband find a jillion things he just can't seem to locate- She takes notes on what he wants her to do before she gets home from work. **(secretary role)** All very quietly, so the kids stay asleep so she can get ready herself.

2. When she is ready and has kissed her husband and waved goodbye to him, she gets the kids up for school, fixes breakfast **(cook role)** and makes sure they look nice, brush their teeth, have their homework packed in their backpacks and then drives them to school. **(chauffer role)**

3. Off to work she goes briefcase in hand. **(career woman)**

4. After she has put in 8-10 hours, she stops by the cleaners to pick up hubby's clothes, the grocery store and then drags herself home- **(gofer role)** Her husband has already picked up the children and is waiting for her at home.

5. But her day isn't over yet- In fact, it's only 50% over. She is greeted at the door with a barrage of vital pieces of information of the day's happenings from every member of the family that must be addressed immediately **(Wizardess of Oz role).** Little Johnny fell on the playground today and skinned his knee so she puts on her Florence Nightingale hat and nurses his little booboo. **(Dr. Mom role)**

6. She changes clothes and starts supper **(cook role).**

7. While supper is cooking, she starts the kids on their homework **(teacher role).** She is amazed at how much teaching she has to do at home.

8. While she is in the kitchen, she notices that the disposal isn't working, so she gets the trusty broomstick and jars it loose! **(handyman role)**

9. After she is finished serving supper and finally gets to eat herself, she does the dishes, straightens the house, does the dusting and puts on a load of laundry **(maid role).**

10. She puts the kids down for bed, 6 times, and then heads for the bed herself. But guess what? Guess who is in the mood for love? You guessed right! Casanova is well rested and ready to put his remote control down and receive some attention. Enter the Siren of Love **(lover role).**

11. She finally gets to sleep- she is the last member of the family to close her eyes and then it starts all over again the next day!

12. On the weekend, she has her yard work to catch up on **(gardener role)** checkbook to balance **(bookkeeper role),** and soccer, basketball or football games to attend **(chauffer & cheerleader role)** or recitals and all the other events that require the attention of what society calls "a good mother".

If this weren't impossible enough, add to her daily responsibilities the full-time job of caregiving for her LO! Exactly where would you cut back, time wise, in the scenario we just painted for you, to squeeze in care for her LO that is completely dependent on her such as:

1. changing diapers
2. bathing
3. filling medication sets
4. doctor appointments
5. dental and eye doctor appointments
6. manicures and pedicures
7. hair appointments
8. interviewing, hiring and re-hiring, training and re-training sitters or live-in help
9. constantly cleaning up one mess after another
10. extra laundry out the kazoo!

Does any of this ring a bell? Are you a paid-up member of The Taffy Trap Club? There are tens of thousands of men and women alike who are members of this special club.

If you *are* a member, please take a bow and then take advantage of the following tips so you can remain emotionally, mentally and physically balanced. You owe it to your LO, your family and especially, to yourself!

22 Creative Tips to Avoid Caregiver Burn-out & Get Control of Your Life Again!

There is a little story I once heard many years ago about a man named Sam who was a workaholic. He would work day and night and some weeks he didn't take a day off and he did this for years.

One day he had a conversation with Pete, a co-worker, who had just gotten back from a two-week vacation in Hawaii.

When Pete told Sam how refreshed he was and how much fun he had with his wife.

Sam said "I wish I could go to Hawaii. I have always wanted to. I have spent the past eleven years dreaming about the waves, the sand, and the ocean breeze. I think about it all the time I am working."

Pete replied "Then why don't you just go. What's stopping you?"

Sam followed Pete's advice and went to Hawaii two months later with his wife. The third day of his vacation, while he was lounging on the beautiful white-sanded beach, breeze blowing in his hair, the sound and sight of the blue-green translucent waves pounding the shore, what do you think was on his mind? You guessed it; the work he wasn't getting done by sitting there in Hawaii!

We must take time for ourselves if we want to be at our best for our family.

The following are our tips to avoid caregiver burnout and show you how to do just that.

PLAN OF ACTION!

TIP # 1:

Forgive yourself and others- for everything. Make a list and cross each offense out with a red pen. This will make the next step much easier.

TIP # 2:

Enlist family and friends to help. The most obvious place to look to for help is your own family. Enlist your siblings or your own children, if you have them, and if they are willing to help.

Learn how to delegate. Make a list of everything that must be done for your LO and then hold a family meeting. Invite all relatives.

Pass the list around and ask each one to write their name next to the task(s) they are willing to take on and then, most importantly- let them do it their way.

You can gently explain how you have been doing it up to now but then let it alone. If you are too pushy, you risk losing their help altogether in the future. Be sure and praise them when they have actually "shown up" and done it too!

TIP # 3:

Ask your friends or neighbors to come and stay with your LO while you go grocery shopping or run your errands.

TIP # 4:

Investigate medical students at the local colleges. Perhaps they need a place to live-in. Check out their references and be sure to talk to their parents and professors before deciding on one.

You can trade room and board for their help sitting with your LO while you get away in addition to getting some help around the house. Be sure to set up the rules and guidelines in a written, signed agreement to avoid future misunderstandings.

TIP # 5:

For at least thirty minutes a day, rest all of your senses. In our bedroom, we have the windows darkened by solid insulation which permits no light to enter in. We have a ceiling fan to keep it cool in addition to our central air. We have a very comfortable bed. Without fail, once a day, I make sure someone is available to tend to our patients so I can retreat to our room, lie down and rest my senses. I use earplugs to block out all sound. (Don't do this unless someone is there to fill in for you)

On occasion, I am able to get a two hour nap! But even if it's only for thirty minutes, I feel refreshed and ready to go again. While you rest, clear your mind. When my mind is on overload, I picture a huge, blank movie screen and concentrate to keep it blank. You may have your own method. Whatever works for you is fine!

TIP # 6:

Hire some help. If financial resources are there, hire a live-in housekeeper. Room and board help to cut down on their weekly pay. Screen them well and check out the last three places they worked to get an idea of their character and skills.

It would be best if you hire someone who has had experience working with the elderly so they aren't stand-off-ish when they need to fill in for you. Make sure that you pay them on time and give them at least one day a week off. If they do not perform well, give them their two weeks' notice and start again.

TIP # 7:

Develop a creative outlet. When family caregivers care for someone who is dying,

many times they feel like it's futile because "soon he will be gone and there is nothing that I can do that will be of any lasting value." This is far from the truth.

How would you feel when he's gone if you didn't do your utmost best to care for him? You are going to know in your heart, years from now, that you provided him with some of the best loved days of his life and a sense of healthy pride will warm you all over just to remember it.

To avoid that feeling of futility, create an outlet for yourself at home. Take the time to do something that you really enjoy doing. If you like to cook, prepare food in large quantities and freeze it for when family and friends will be coming over.

TIP # 8:

If your LO still enjoys eating, prepare his favorites. Cook for your friends or family in exchange for their coming over to stay so you can get out for a while.

TIP # 9:

If you like gardening, take your portable baby monitor outside with you and do some planting or re-potting.

TIP # 10:

If you've long ago abandoned your painting or drawing because of raising the kids or your career took up all of your time, pick it up again. This is a terrific outlet. If you are good at faces and bodies, paint or draw your LO from his last photo before he got sick. Talk about therapeutic!

TIP # 11:

Maybe you enjoy writing. Keep a diary of your caregiving journey or write that book you've always had in you but didn't have the time to do it. There are many things you can do to stimulate the creativity God put inside you. You will feel fulfilled when you balance this enormous caregiving responsibility with your own need to express that creative spirit.

TIP # 12:

Don't hold back the tears or the laughter. Did you ever see the movie "Steel Magnolias"? (if you didn't, rent it) Remember in the last scene when Sally Fields was sobbing but then without warning, started laughing uncontrollably at her daughter's funeral. It was so real.

Every day, we find a jillion things to laugh at while caregiving for the terminally ill. We laugh at ourselves; humans are really funny if you stop and think about it! Give yourself permission to have some fun. No one will think you are cold or calloused because you don't get up every day and put on sackcloth and ashes. If they do then that's their problem- don't make it yours.

TIP # 13:

When you feel like crying, cry. If you feel the need to have someone hold you while you cry, ask them. How will you know if you are crying "too much"? When minutes of crying turn into hours and then into days and you aren't able to concentrate enough to care for your LO, then you need to seek help. Make an appointment to see your pastor and tell him how you are feeling. He will pray with you and help you get through this.

TIP # 14:

Attend church. Try and get away to go to church. If no one will stay with your LO on Sunday mornings, go on Wednesday nights. See if a family member will go with you. Spiritual support will be the primary key to helping you experience hope for the future.

TIP # 15:

Tap into volunteer services in your area. If your LO is on hospice or has a home health agency, make an appointment with his social worker to discuss any concerns you may have regarding his care and any volunteer services that might be available to sit for you.

TIP # 16:

Take care of your own health:

- Go for a morning walk daily. This will get you out of the house and give you a fresh new perspective on life.
- Get plenty of sleep at night or if your LO has his days and nights mixed up, sleep during the day while he does.
- Watch out for the caffeine trap though. That won't help you. It'll just make you nervous in the long run.
- Know yourself well

enough to guard your alcohol intake. It's not that difficult for you to go from having a drink occasionally to having one or more daily just to numb your senses from the pain you're feeling. If you drink for this reason, you will end up justifying it until you become an alcoholic before you can say lickety-split.

- Take your medications being sure not to skip doses if you are on any. You can't be a good caregiver to your LO if your own health suffers.

TIP # 17:

Join a support group. You may not be able to picture yourself attending a support group but reconsider it. You will be surrounded by other family care-givers going through many of the same situations and experiencing emotions much like yours. They may have discovered ways of coping that never occurred to you.

TIP # 18:

Swap out sitting. If your LO isn't bed-bound yet and is able to leave the house with help, you could develop a few friendships with people who would be willing to swap out a day with you now and then.

You could take your LO over to their house for them to watch in exchange for them coming over to yours. Or, if your LO is bed-bound, you could make a similar arrangement with someone whose LO is still able to travel and you could sit for them in your home and then they could come to yours to help you out. It's worth the

effort. Stretch your borders and rediscover the outside world!

TIP # 19:

Pamper yourself! A minimum of once a week, treat yourself to a facial. Apply it just before you soak in a tub filled with hot, scented water, light some candles and put on soft instrumentals to play in the background. Don't feel guilty pampering yourself while your LO is lying in the next room. You deserve a little time to yourself. Not only do you deserve it, you need it.

TIP # 20:

Start pulling your own strings. Every time the doorbell or phone rings, you do not have to break your neck answering it. Start planning to group your calls and return your messages at one particular timeslot daily. Many times, we are our worst enemy when it comes to time management.

TIP # 21:

Make a list of your goals, obstacles that could come up to prevent you from reaching your goals in each area, what you can do if they do come up to continue toward achieving them, a date in the future of attainment.

Make an appt. with yourself and KEEP IT! Write down everything you want to accomplish. Categories such as spiritual, financial, marital, health, social, acquisitions, children, outlets for creativity. You'll find that if you attain some of your goals every month, the caregiving will go much smoother. You will stop feeling as though you are wasting your life.

Now, place monthly calendars for the next 6 months in front of you on a table. Don't make the huge mistake of planning too much in one week or month. At the end of 6 months, you can accomplish all of it if you plan realistically. Spread out this extra activity, outside of your numerous established routines, and give yourself plenty of lee-way. Bob taught me a long time ago that the only way to eat an elephant is a bite at a time.

TIP # 22:

A date night once a week keeps you young at heart. Leave the kids at home if you are married. If single, go out with your friends to a movie or to your favorite restaurant and let someone else do the cooking for a change.

We have given you many tips in this section to help you plan a rewarding caregiver's relief plan. Don't just read them. Implement them in this season of your life and when you have emerged from it, you will be the richer for doing so.

Depression & Isolation

There can be several reasons the family caregiver becomes depressed and pushes everyone away from them, only to retreat into a solitary existence. If you find yourself in this condition, see if any of the following are some of your reasons. If so, the tips follow the descriptions. (These terms refer to caregiving emotions)

1. Hopelessness: *despair with no solution in sight*

Many times we feel hopeless because we only focus on the problem and then become paralyzed which prevents us from moving on to the solution.

Sit down and write out your action plan for handling whatever situation is depressing you. You'll need a piece of paper, a pen and a calendar with little squares to fill in. First, describe on paper what you are feeling right now.

After you write it all out, read it and pinpoint the problem and put it into one sentence or better yet, into one word. Look in the index in the back of this book for that topic and follow the tips, making a plan to resolve the issue. If you can change the situation, set a date to begin and follow the schedule you have created. Don't put it off.

2. Guilt: *feeling you are somehow to blame*

If this is your main problem, the best advice I have for you is to get my book, *"The Caring Caregivers Guide to Dealing with Guilt."* The book is filled with true stories of 9 different types of guilt that I identified in the course of caring for our elderly over 18 years and excellent, practical tips on slaying the "guilt monster." It is written specifically for caregiver guilt and I believe it will help you to resolve this destructive and paralyzing emotion. There are too many tips to include in this section so my best tip regarding guilt is to buy the book. You can order it from the form in the back of this book.

3. Apathy: *the state of a lack of responsiveness, responsibility, concern or interest*

You feel this way, subconsciously, when you are trying to protect yourself from further heartache. You give up because you don't see any point in carrying on. You have been overwhelmed with work, emotion or responsibility. This is one of the major signs of burnout. As a caregiver, this can become dangerous to your LO in regard to their care needs.

If you recognize this description or the symptoms, it is imperative that you have a relative or friend come to stay with you for a week or two to relieve you of your caregiving duties. When you have someone to stay with your LO, choose several options from the caregiver burnout section of this book. If you don't act, you may find yourself sinking down deeper and deeper into depression until it's practically impossible to find yourself again.

Apathy must be tackled head-on and the fact that you are reading this book shows that you still have some concern left for yourself or your LO.

4. Grief: *sorrow, heartache or anguish*

When we are young, we think our parents will live forever. When we fall in love and marry, we can't imagine that some day we will be alone due to their dying. How many times have spouses said, "Either I'm going first or we are going together!" But it doesn't happen that way, does it? One is usually left behind to carry on and it can be devastatingly lonely to do so.

There is also loss before death. Your parent or spouse filled a very important role in your life and now these roles have been changed. You miss the former relationship.

If your LO has been diagnosed with Alzheimer's disease, he will "look" the same on the outside but his behavior will become radically and irreversibly changed as he deteriorates. Friends and many relatives may not understand your grief due to a lack of knowledge in this area, not realizing that it is a terminal disease. This can make it extremely difficult for you to cope with.

You really need to seek out a support group made up of other

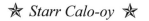

family members going through the same thing you are. Listen to them and you won't feel so isolated anymore. The facilitators usually bring in some wonderfully informative speakers to educate the attendees and answer questions.

5. Lack of concentration: *inability to focus*

Believe it or not, you can control what you think about. Your mind may be like a little puppy, jumping on your legs and running around, but with a little practice, you can leash your thoughts to obey your will.

We were designed by God to think of only one thing at a time. Allow me to prove it: Think of a huge, pink elephant. Were you thinking of anything else as you read that? Okay, now, don't think of a yellow kangaroo. What did you just picture? I rest my case.

If you are dwelling on all of your problems, start replacing those thoughts with the solutions. You need to write them down and keep the list with you at all times. It will take some self-discipline, but you can do it.

6. Fatigue: *exhaustion and a general lack of energy*

Very simply put, get some shut-eye! Read the chapter on "Outside help" and put one of those tips into motion. Bob has always said "Fatigue makes cowards of us all." If you have trouble falling to sleep, read the chapter on "ZZZZ's" and follow those tips.

7. Fear: *worry that turns into panic*

There are numerous fears but let's focus on common caregiver fears here. There is the fear of facing the death of your LO, fear of being alone and fear of losing touch with who you were before the caregiving started.

If your LO has a terminal illness and is on hospice service, ask the case manager to set up an appointment with the Chaplain to meet with you at your home. The hospice chaplains specialize in all of the emotional issues revolving around death so this can be a perfect match. There is no charge for this vitally important service provided by your hospice. You do not have to ride this emotional roller coaster alone.

8. Unforgiveness & Resentment: *blame, condemnation, accusations & bitterness*

Forgiveness is a choice- not a feeling. Do you smell with your eyes? Do you hear with your tongue? Well, you don't "feel" forgiveness either. Once you decide to forgive someone, it might be lip service at first, but soon it will become a reality in your life.

Also, your forgiveness of someone who has offended you does not depend on their repentance. Jesus forgave the very people He created as they were killing Him. So, if your LO's state of mind does not provide the ability to hold an intelligent, lucid conversation, do not use this as an excuse to hold on to the past and not forgive them for what they did or didn't do to you.

If you choose not to forgive, it will only tear you apart the rest of your life. It hurts you more than it hurts them. It's like drinking poison yourself and expecting them to die!

How do you forgive? Sit down alone and make a list of everything your LO has done to you over the course of your life. Don't leave anything out. Next, get a red marker and cross out each offense as you say out loud:

"I make a decision to forgive <u>(the name of the person)</u> for <u>(describe the offence)</u>. I do not feel forgiveness in my heart right now but I know that my heavenly Father will not forgive me if I do not forgive others, so I choose to forgive."

As you use the red marker, it signifies that the blood of Jesus covers all sin. Once you have done this, it won't be long before you feel better; about yourself and about your LO. Choose to actively not remember their sin against you. Every time it comes up in your mind, purposely think about something else- don't take it back. You will make progress and overcome.

CAREGIVER ILLNESS & DEATH

The overwhelming stress of caring for a chronically or terminally ill LO can cause you, the family caregiver, to be highly susceptible to illness themselves and can lead to premature death. Therefore, it is imperative that plans are made far in advance for alternative care for your LO.

Even if you get the common flu or a cold, it can be life

threatening to an elderly person. When we cared for the elderly in our own home, we would not allow anyone who was ill to enter our home. If any one of our family got sick, we would put them in quarantine so the virus would not infect others and they did not come out of the room until they were completely well.

The time to put the following tips into practice is as soon as you become a caregiver.

PLAN OF ACTION!

TIP # 1:

Start a care notebook with section tabs as follows:

- Emergency contacts (alternate caregiver contact information,
- Doctors
- Insurances
- Pastor/rabbi/priest
- Police department
- Family members-list all cell, home and work phone numbers.
- My LOs behavior (this should have a detailed description of his behavioral problems and what you have found to be helpful in dealing with him. Keep this section updated as he changes)
- Medications (List all medications he is currently taking along with the time of day he takes them and the dosage. Also, write the pharmacy information and insurance company here. Very important: update this regularly including an archive history of what didn't work for him so that the person who takes over for you won't repeat it.)
- Sleeping, eating and exercise habits and routines.
- Legal Issues (Place

pocketed folders in this section clearly marked and containing the location of his will, living will, banking information, and any other legal paperwork you have gathered after reading the "Paperwork" chapter.

You can add sections as you go along. Keep this notebook visible and make sure that trusted family members know about it in case they are contacted.

TIP # 2:

It would be wise to enlist at least two alternate caregivers. They should be people you trust with your personal possessions, money, and the care of your LO. They need to have empathy, compassion, be in relatively good health and an earnest desire to protect your LOs rights and maintain their dignity. They need to know about the care notebook and be willing to come immediately in the event of an emergency.

TIP # 3:

If you don't have a phone with speed dialing options, get one and then program it to dial your alternate caregivers, EMS, 911, police, fire department, all doctors and trusted family members. Place a list of the speed dial digits, in large letters and numbers on the walls of your home in strategic locations so if you are incapacitated, you can easily see them.

TIP # 4:

Get a cell phone and keep it on your person at all times. Program it with speed dial emergency numbers (listed above).

TIP # 5:

Plan out your funeral and make all funeral

arrangements. See an attorney and have him draw up your will, living will and select an administrator of your estate and a medical and financial power of attorney for you. Make sure that trusted family members know your wishes and the location of the contact information for your attorney and doctors.

TIP # 6:

Do not cover up your LO's illness. It would be devastating for your family to suddenly find out that your LO was terminally ill and that they had the responsibility for taking over their care.

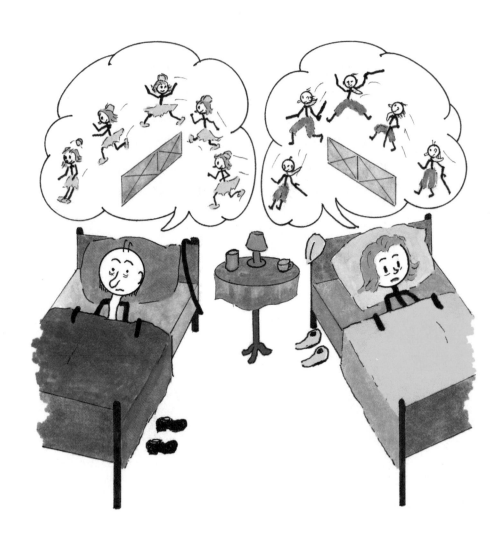

I Didn't Sleep at All Last Night

ᴵZᴵ

ZZZZ'S

THIS CHAPTER:

- **The Family Caregiver's Sleep**
- **Sleeping Tips for Your LO**

ZZZZ'S

Let's talk about sleep difficulties. Most of the books we have all read on caregiving focus on the patient's rest, but <u>your</u> time-out is of the utmost importance. Without it, your ability to be a caring caregiver with someone's very life in your hands becomes greatly encumbered.

Just a few of the areas effected greatly by a lack of sleep are:

1) **Your concentration level- which can alter the level of care you provide**
2) **Irritability- loss of patience**
3) **Resentment of the situation- which can lead to abuse**
4) **Immunity to illnesses goes down**
5) **Depression- which can lead to neglect**
6) **Memory trouble- which can put your LO in harm's way**

THE FAMILY CAREGIVER'S SLEEP

PLAN OF ACTION!

TIP # 1:

Get into your bed when you are ready to go to sleep. Do not watch television in bed. Do not eat in bed. Do not read in bed and do not work in bed. Retrain your brain to view your bed as a place to go to sleep. You will soon be looking forward to climbing in and pulling the covers over your head.

TIP # 2:

Start using wax earplugs but make sure someone in the house keeps an ear out for activity during the night. Make sure your room is dark. If you use a fan directly on you, you will sleep better. Your brain gets used to the sound of the fan and being so cool, snuggling under the covers, that you easily go to sleep. How do we know this? We do it and have no problem at all!

TIP # 3:

Go to Home Depot and buy some lightweight silver-coated Styrofoam insulation, cut it to fit the inside of your bedroom

windows and place them in there. Now, you can take a nap with your earplugs and fan during the day when you have someone to watch over your LO.

Caregivers have to be up late at night many times a week so it is imperative to nap during the day. If you are too tired from being awake too long, you will have trouble sleeping at night. If you can nap during the day soundly, you will sleep better at night.

Doesn't sound logical because we try to keep our babies awake all day so they will sleep at night but we aren't babies. Our sleep cycles are much different and we work, babies do not.

If you will allow all of your senses to rest; to completely shut down every day, you will not only sleep better, you will be happier and calmer.

TIP # 4:

Eat a light supper; stay away from alcohol; stay away from caffeine and sugar, allow yourself to gradually wind down before attempting to sleep and do not get in bed until you're sleepy.

TIP # 5:

As a last resort, talk to your doctor about something to help you sleep at night. Ask him for something that doesn't leave you feeling drugged in the morning and is not addictive. You may have to experiment with the time you take it at night so you sleep all night long. Be sure not to take more than prescribed. Some medications take time to get into your system, so if you feel it is not working, call your doctor and get his recommendations before you make any changes.

SLEEPING TIPS FOR YOUR LO

PLAN OF ACTION!

TIP # 1:

Put a nightlight in their room and either a bedside commode (if they are not in diapers) or a nightlight in the hall and bathroom, to light their way, if they still are able to get up and toilet themselves. If not…

TIP # 2:

…Put an open intercom or baby monitor in their room, and put the mate for it next to your bed.

TIP # 3:

Make sure your LO takes an early afternoon nap. If they will not lie down, try lying down with them on their bed and snuggling. Tell them that you need to be held like they held you as a child and that you cannot go to sleep without their arms. Have soft music on low and you may get faster results.

TIP # 4:

If your LO is not in jeopardy of falling and wants to pace or wander all through the house, let them. When they finally get tired,

suggest they rest. Portable gates can help keep them out of unsafe areas. All you have to do is secure them a little higher than you would for a baby or use two in the door jamb rather than one.

TIP # 5:

Try keeping a television on low volume at night, all night, but not on anything violent. Try a Christian network. The voices and low light may be just what your LO needs to help them start sleeping longer periods.

TIP # 6:

Make sure his bedding is comfortable. We found that using comforters rather than sheets and bedspreads worked much better. Sheets tend to tangle more easily.

TIP # 7:

Check to see if your LO is too hot or cold and adjust the room temperature accordingly.

TIP # 8:

Use darkening blinds on windows to keep intruding security or street lights out of their eyes at night and to block out the bright, morning sunlight.

TIP # 9:

As a last resort, ask your doctor for something to help your LO sleep at night. Give it to them as late as possible so its effects will last. Do not expect them to sleep more than six hours at a time in the early stages of dementia. In later stages they will sleep more than they are awake.

TIP # 10:

At least thirty minutes before you tuck him in, make sure everything is peaceful and quiet and that you speak more softly to him than you usually do during the day. In time, he will begin to associate this routine with bedtime and wind down more readily.

TIP # 11:

Try a mild massage with some mineral oil mixed with lavender lotion. Heat the mixture before you begin. Do not talk while you perform the massage. Play some calming ocean sounds or nature music as you massage. Keep the lighting very low. Keep your LO warm and covered as you go. Massage slowly and gently and when you are through, kiss him good night and leave the room.

INDEX

INDEX

C

D

E

F

G

J

K

L

M

334

T

V

W

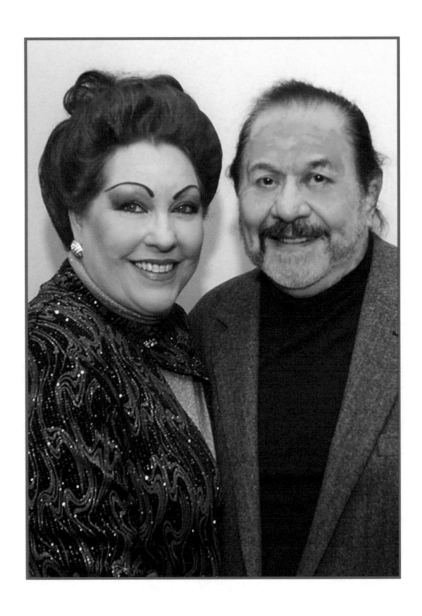

The Authors

Starr & Bob Calo-oy

About the Authors: Starr & Bob Calo-oy
"Caregiving Tips A-Z,
Alzheimer's & Other Dementias"

Bob & Starr Calo-oy were both born and raised in San Antonio and have been joyfully married for 27 years. From 1989 to 2006, they owned and operated a personal care home specializing in the care of terminally ill patients and victims of Alzheimer's disease and other forms of dementia in their San Antonio home. They also cared for the well-minded elderly who could no longer care for themselves at home.

In addition to caring for the elderly in their home, they have given in-service training for doctors, nurses, the staffs of hospices and home health agencies, sharing tips and unique ideas for caring for people with dementia. Starr also gives private consultations to individuals on how to start and operate a successful personal care home as well as helping family caregivers set up their home for care.

She is a columnist for SAWorship.com as well as an occasional freelance writer for the San Antonio Express-News.

In April 2004, they released their first book, *"The Caring Caregivers Guide to Dealing with Guilt",* about their experiences over 18 years of operating their personal care home. This book is about the undeserved guilt families experience when they turn the care of their loved ones over to someone else. However, if the family desires to care for their loved one in their own home, it provides tips and directions to help them. It was written so that the medical field can benefit by empathizing while at the same time making it easy for the non-medical professional to easily understand its content.

In November 2006, they released *"Hospice Care at Home/ A guide to caring for your dying loved one at home."* This book provides the family caregiver with all the information necessary to keep their loved one in their home through death rather than sending them to a more institutional setting. It has sold over 2,000 copies over the past few months and is on its way to becoming a best seller. This book is now available in Spanish also.

In November 2007, they released 2 books:

- *"Caregiving Tips A-Z, Alzheimer's & Other Dementias"*
- *"Caregiving Tips A-Z"*

These books will be available in Spanish in March 2008.

Starr and Bob published their own monthly, 26-page tabloid newspaper, the **TELESTARR**, which was circulated throughout South Texas city, county and state agencies for eight years.

Presently, they counsel couples to help them to develop a more meaningful relationship and better communication skills.

In September, 2007, they started the non-profit organization, Caregivers Support Network, through which they will begin teaching free caregiving classes in February 2008 which will be open to the public.

Starr and Bob speak at conventions, seminars, civic clubs, and health care facilities, do book signings at Barnes & Noble's all over Texas, and make television and radio appearances.

Elder Rage by Jacqueline Marcell
Order Form

Fax　(949) 975-1013 *(Tear out and fax this form)*
Phone　(949) 975-1012 *(Have your credit card ready)*
Internet　www.ElderRage.com. See: ORDER HERE
　　　　Email: jmarcell@elderrage.com
Mail　Send this form with a check, or your credit card info to:
　　　　Impressive Press
　　　　3141 Michelson Dr., Suite 606
　　　　Irvine, California 92612-5670

Please send _____ copies of the Impressive Press book

Elder Rage by Jacqueline Marcell
(Please Print CLEARLY)

Company

Name

Address

City　　　　　**St**　　　**Zip**

Phone (　　)

Email

CA Sales Tax: Add 7.75% for books shipped within California
Example: One book: 24.95 + 1.94 Sales Tax = $26.89 (*plus* shipping)

Shipping: US: Add $4 for the first book and $3 for each additional

Total: $_____ ❑ Check enclosed *(Sorry, no COD)*

To Order by Credit Card *(Please check one)*

❑ Visa　　❑ American Express　　❑ MasterCard

Name on Card

Account Number

Expiration Date

Signature

Comments

443

Elder Rage by Jacqueline Marcell
Order Form

Fax　(949) 975-1013 *(Tear out and fax this form)*
Phone　(949) 975-1012 *(Have your credit card ready)*
Internet　www.ElderRage.com. See: ORDER HERE
　　　　Email: jmarcell@elderrage.com
Mail　Send this form with a check, or your credit card info to:
　　　　Impressive Press
　　　　3141 Michelson Dr., Suite 606
　　　　Irvine, California 92612-5670

Please send _____ copies of the Impressive Press book

Elder Rage by Jacqueline Marcell
(Please Print CLEARLY)

Company _____

Name _____

Address _____

City _____ **St** _____ **Zip** _____

Phone (_____ **)** _____

Email _____

CA Sales Tax: Add 7.75% for books shipped within California
Example: One book: 24.95 + 1.94 Sales Tax = $26.89 (***plus*** shipping)

Shipping: US: Add $4 for the first book and $3 for each additional

Total: $_____ ❑ Check enclosed *(Sorry, no COD)*

To Order by Credit Card *(Please check one)*
❑ Visa　　❑ American Express　　❑ MasterCard

Name on Card _____

Account Number _____

Expiration Date _____

Signature _____

Comments _____

444

Books by Starr & Bob Calo-oy
Order Form

Fax   (210) 979-0900
Phone (210) 521-8668 *(Have your credit card ready)*
Internet www.caregiversadvice.net See: BOOKSTORE
      Email: starrcalo-oy@satx.rr.com
Mail Send this form with a check, or your credit card info to:
      Orchard Publications
      6619 Laurel Hill
      San Antonio, Texas 78229

Please send _____ copies of the Orchard Publications book ($29.95)
***Caregiving Tips A-Z* by Starr & Bob Calo-oy**
Please send _____ copies of the Orchard Publications book ($14.95)
***Hospice Care at Home* by Starr & Bob Calo-oy**
Please send _____ copies of the Orchard Publications book ($14.95)
***The Caring Caregivers Guide to Dealing with Guilt* by Starr & Bob Calo-oy**
Please send _____ copies of the Orchard Publications book ($29.95)
***Caregiving Tips A-Z, Alzheimer's & Other Dementias* by Starr & Bob Calo-oy**

(Please Print CLEARLY)

Name _____

Address _____

City _____**St** _____**Zip** _____

Phone (**)** _____

Email _____

TX Sales Tax: Add 8.25% for books shipped within Texas
Example: One tip book: $29.95 + $2.47 Sales Tax = $32.42 (*plus* shipping)

Shipping: US: Add $5 for the first book and $4 for each additional

Total: $_____ ☐ Check enclosed *(Sorry, no COD)*

To Order by Credit Card *(Please check one)*

☐ Visa   ☐ American Express   ☐ MasterCard

Name on Card _____

Account Number _____

Expiration Date _____

Signature _____

DATE DUE

GAYLORD   PRINTED IN U.S.A.